Sperm Donor Offspring:
Identity and Other Experiences

Visit www.booksurge.com to order additional copies.

LYNNE W SPENCER

SPERM DONOR OFFSPRING:

IDENTITY AND OTHER EXPERIENCES

2007

Sperm Donor Offspring:
Identity and Other Experiences

TABLE OF CONTENTS

ABSTRACT

Sperm Donor Offspring: Identity and Other Experiences is derived from my thesis at the Center for Humanistic Studies (now the Michigan School of Professional Psychology) for my Master of Arts in Humanistic and Clinical Psychology in the year 2000. The research is a qualitative phenomenological exploration titled "What is the experience of confronting the reality of being a donor offspring?" i.e., a person who was conceived using donor sperm. There is little research from the perspective of the donor offspring regarding their experience. This study validates and expands upon previous research on the experience of donor offspring. Eight donor offspring were interviewed, in person or by phone, using a few biographical questions followed by an open ended format allowing the full range of their experience of confronting the reality of being a donor offspring to be explored. Research participants ranged in age from 39 to 57. The age of being informed of being a donor offspring ranged from 18 to 47. Four were male and four were female. Five were conceived in the United States, and three were conceived in the United Kingdom. The themes of donor offspring involved feelings regarding secrecy, feeling different, doubt about paternity, feeling of not fitting in their family, identity confusion, search for the sperm donor and need for ancestral connection, feeling a connection with half-siblings, concern about the next generation and inherited medical conditions, feeling alone, having a need for support and information, finding support and similar experiences in adoption groups, an array of strong feelings, wanting to normalize being a donor offspring and accept the reality, developing beliefs that knowledge of genetic and medical history is a birthright, finding a sense of purpose and speaking up about the experience of being a donor offspring. The experience of donor offspring is relevant for personal, clinical, educational, societal, policy and regulation related to donor insemination and other reproductive technologies. Now that there are a significant number of adolescent and adult donor offspring, research on their experience is important in defining the practice of donor insemination.

To Cheryl, Liz, and Nicole, thank you for entering my life, and being the amazing souls that you are.

To my parents, for wanting children enough to pursue donor insemination. To my mom, for telling the truth.

To Karen, for sharing the journey with me.

To Mike K., thank you for believing in me as I confronted my reality of being a donor offspring and for teaching me that I am a pioneer in life.

To Bill, donor support groups, donor offspring, families, counselors, and all who have explored the journey of donor conception, for supporting me and many others along the way.

To the Center for Humanistic Studies (currently the Michigan School of Professional Psychology), Matt, and Sandi, for promoting humanism in life, for being authentic, for clinical and spiritual guidance, and for supporting our healing journeys.

"In all of us there is a hunger marrow deep to know our heritage, to know who we are and from where we have come from. Without this enriching knowledge, there is a hollow yearning, no matter what our attainments in life there is a most disquieting loneliness."

ROOTS
Alex Haley

CHAPTER I
PERSONAL KNOWLEDGE AND EXPERIENCE

I was walking with my mom in the mall. My dad had just died a few days earlier, and I was still in town. My mom said, "There's something I have to tell you..." Long pause..."Your father may not have been your real father." She told me that I was conceived through artificial insemination. The doctor had mixed sperm from my dad and an anonymous donor, so my parents never knew if my father was my biological father. All of a sudden, a lot of things in my life made sense. I felt a great sense of relief.

This is the beginning of my research thesis question. My conception through donor insemination, and living in a family formed in this way, was the foundation of my life. Finding out about the sperm donor was the beginning of my awareness of my true identity. This situation brings me to the research question I chose to study. What is the experience of confronting the reality of being a donor offspring?

In confronting the reality of my new knowledge, my first goal was to find out who my biological father was. We did DNA tests—using a tissue sample the hospital had of my dad, and blood samples from my mom, sister, and I, and found out scientifically that indeed my father was not my genetic father. My genetic father was an anonymous sperm donor, and my sister and I are full genetic sisters. We had the same sperm donor.

I have two fathers. The father I grew up with was my "dad". My biological father is an anonymous sperm donor, the man who Dr. Trythall found to donate sperm to my parents, half of my genetic foundation.

What was the motivation of this sperm donor? Did he just want to make a few bucks to get through medical school? Was he altruistic in giving my parents and myself the gift of life? Did he want to spread his genetic material in the world?

Who is this genetic father of mine? He is probably a doctor, probably graduated from Wayne State University Medical School in Detroit in the late 1950's, should have brown eyes, probably has type A blood, and that's about all I know. Dr. Trythall is dead, so I can't seek information from him. The doctors who bought Dr. Trythall's practice and records won't tell me anything about my sperm donor. Is he a nice person? Does he have a family of his own? Is he honest with them? How many donor offspring did he have? How many half-blood siblings do I have? What is his ethnic background? What is half of my ethnic background? Am I partly Native American after all? Or am I partly Italian? Greek? Eastern European? Is he shy? Is my shyness genetic? What other parts of me are prescribed by my genes? What parts of me do I share in likeness with this man?

I wonder how he perceives having been a sperm donor. Does he ever even think about it? Does he ever wonder who his genetic offspring are? Does he have any concern for them?

I am the sperm donor's "offspring", his genetic child. I have tried to find him. I don't want money or an inheritance from him. I can't expect to have an ongoing relationship with him. But in the core of my being, I want to know who he is. I want to see him. I want to know what that half of my ethnic background is. I want to know what his interests, hobbies, mannerisms, and quirks are, and if I have any of the same. I wonder why I became a nurse, and considered becoming a physician, when nobody else in my family was in the medical field. Is there a genetic link to my interests?

Wondering is part of being a donor offspring for me. Since I don't have answers to some of the questions of my life, I can only wonder what the truth is.

After considering the meaning to me of being a donor's offspring, I began to wonder, shouldn't I have the right to know my origins? If my life belongs to me, shouldn't I be able to know what my ethnic background is? Shouldn't I be able to know who my genetic father is? If my life is for other people's purposes, and not my own, then what is the purpose of my life?

These are some of the questions and struggles that I went through with confronting a life of deceit. For myself, I just want the truth. I just want the missing pieces of my identity. I feel that my identity should be my rightful property, not owned by doctors.

My foundation had been knocked out from under me. I had to rebuild my sense of self, my identity. For me, confronting the reality of being a donor offspring was a process of healing. It involved looking back at the meaning of events in my life and looking at the relationships in my life. It involved finding a way to move on, reclaiming my voice and my life, and working towards my life's purpose.

I chose to do my thesis research on the reality of being a donor offspring. How do other donor offspring confront the reality of this situation? What is their experience?

Some themes for me related to confronting the reality of being a donor offspring were: What is the meaning of personal identity? How much is it related to nature v. nurture? What is the meaning of trust in relationships? What is acceptance or non-acceptance (unconditional or conditional love) of a child in a family created in this way, even when they are different from others in the family? How is sexuality viewed and talked about in the family? What is the social atmosphere like in the family? What is the nature of the relationships in the family? What is the relationship of an anonymous sperm donor and his "donor offspring"? Does the donor offspring feel a sense of abandonment? I wanted to find out if my experiences in understanding and confronting being a donor offspring are similar to other donor offspring. What are the themes for other people with this experience?

In Chapter I, I have shared some of my experiences as a donor offspring and confronting this reality in my life. After writing about my own experience, I conducted the thesis research, interviewing other donor offspring about their experience confronting the reality of being a donor offspring. I have used a phenomenological research model to determine the themes of this experience.

In the process of adapting this thesis research into book form, I have chosen to leave the majority of the description about the research process in the document. It gives a bigger picture of how this information was developed. Some readers may not care to read about the details of this process and they can skip forward to Chapter VI to find out the results of what donor offspring identified as important in their experience of confronting the reality of being donor offspring.

Chapters II and III involve preparing for the thesis study. In Chapter II, I define the terms of my thesis research question to focus and narrow it, and make it more clear. Chapter III is a literature review to look at other related research studies and find the fit of this thesis study in the framework of what has previously been done.

The phenomenological model and the research methods used are described in chapters IV and V of this study. The guiding interview questions I focused on are in Appendix F.

In Chapter VI, I present the data from interviews with other donor offspring. Finally, in Chapter VII, I discuss the implications and applications of the study of the experience of confronting the reality of being a donor offspring.

CHAPTER II
STATEMENT OF THE RESEARCH QUESTION

Out of my personal experience has come an interest, and indeed passion, for understanding the effects of donor insemination on the people involved: the parents, the offspring, the donor, the physician and other medical personnel, and the people that they connect with. I considered doing research with sperm donors in order to see what their experience was, especially in terms of how being a sperm donor affects the relationships in their lives. After deep consideration and reaching out to people, I realized that it would be difficult for me to find sperm donors willing to participate in this type of study. I am outside of their circle of connections, and due to the historically secret nature of being a sperm donor, the private nature of this phenomenological study would be challenging.

Initially, I was leery of doing my research from the point of view of the donor offspring. I have heard many heart-wrenching stories of the circumstances of donor offspring. This brings up feelings for me related to being victimized and not in control of parts of one's life. I was afraid of hearing this pain from people as I have before. After further exploration, and having my own pain resurface, I knew that the viewpoint of the donor offspring was important for others to hear, and for me in continuing along my healing journey.

My thesis question started as "What is the experience of being a donor offspring?" My thesis advisor felt this was not specific enough to study qualitatively. We explored concepts together, and redefined it as "What is the experience of coming to terms with being a donor offspring?" The goal was to delineate a particular experience in time, as opposed to something which is always a part of a person's identity.

In preparing my thesis proposal, I became uncomfortable with the concept of "coming to terms." It felt passive. I felt a sense of resignation. It implies that we come to an end in our journey. We get there. I do not feel an end to this journey for myself, that I have come to terms with being a donor offspring. I have learned to live my life without being centered around this aspect of my life, but my pain reminded me that the journey has not ended.

I began to wonder how to redefine this study in a manner of getting to the heart of the experience. How does an individual feel about being a donor offspring? What emotions do they experience? What are their felt sensations in their body when contemplating being a donor offspring? What do they think about? What are their perceptions of the experience? How do they react or interact with other people in their lives around this aspect of themselves? How do they react behaviorally in relation to being a donor offspring?

I decided to study donor offspring who have actively pursued the meaning of being donor offspring in their lives. These are people who have reached out to others to talk about this experience, to find support, and to offer support to others. I wanted to study people who have persevered in their process of relating to being a donor offspring to explore its infinite possibilities, and who have shared their perceptions with others. I wanted to interview people who have taken action on their experience of being a donor offspring and brought it out to the world at large. I wanted to explore the experience of people who have actively confronted the fact of being a donor offspring and shared this reality with others.

As a result, my question evolved to be "What is the experience of confronting the reality of being a donor offspring?" In this chapter, I define the words in this question to further delineate what is to be studied.

In human science qualitative research such as this, a particular sector of the experience of being human is studied. Carl Rogers (1980), in describing experience and the creation of meaning, states "at all times there is going on in the human organism a flow of experiencings to which the individual can turn again and again as a referent in order to discover the meaning of those experiences" (p. 141). This is what qualitative human research participants are asked to do: to explore the experience again and again, in order to get to the themes, the descriptions, and the meaning of the particular experience.

The term "co-researcher" is part of the framework of qualitative research. By its nature, it shows the central importance of the research participant in defining the study. The co-researcher, or research participant, is allowed an open-ended exploration of the topic. Whatever is important for them in this experience is what becomes a theme of the research study.

In describing one woman's experience, Rogers (1980) states:
When she could be open to all her experiencing-both her inner experiencing, and her experiencing of the demands and attitudes of others-she would have a basis by which to live. She would discover that her experiencing, if she could be open to it and could listen sensitively for its meaning, would provide a constructive guide for her behavior and for her life....She could discover that it was safe to communicate her self more completely. She would discover that she did not need to be lonely and isolated, that another could understand and share the meaning of her experience. (pp. 177-178)

This points out not only the meaning in our experiencing but also the importance of reaching out to others and sharing our personal experience. Experience is the basis for humanistic qualitative research.

I have come to appreciate the need to "confront the reality" of being a donor offspring. It is an intense, multifaceted experience. Being a donor offspring is a reality of one's life, not something which one can choose or not choose, or make changes to. If a person is a donor offspring, that is a reality for that person. It is his or her truth.

The Dictionary of Psychology (Corsini, 1999) defines a "reality confrontation" as "a situation occurring when new and correct information is presented that differs from prior beliefs or opinions, as in a child learning that the couple thought to be biological parents actually adopted the child" (p.809). Similarly, with donor offspring, after holding prior beliefs that their social fathers are also their biological fathers, it is sometimes learned that in actuality, a sperm donor is their biological father. The donor offspring must then confront what consciously is a new reality, but what was an actual reality all along. In some cases, donor offspring grow up knowing their biological father is a sperm donor, but still must confront the reality of what that means for them in their lives.

To me, confronting a reality implies an active process. Berenson and Mitchell (1974) also express this view. They describe confrontation as an active, evaluative response, and as a response to discrepancies. Confrontations encourage a person "to act upon his world in some reasonable, appropriate and constructive manner, and discouraging a passive stance toward life" (p. iii). When there is a discrepancy, in this case between the former knowledge and new learned knowledge about the status of a person's biological father, acting upon his or her world in some manner follows, if one confronts the experience. Adler and Myerson (1991) concur. According to them, confrontation involves getting a person's "attention, producing a reaction in him, and demanding that he change.... A confrontation is aimed at unmasking denial" (p.11).

One final definition which is important is that of "donor offspring." Terminology has been difficult in this field. Historically, in legal cases, donor offspring have been referred to as "semiadopted" and "not illegitimate" (Noble, 1987, p. 261), or "semi-bastard" (Schellen, 1957, p. 303). The social father was called the "foster-father" (Schellen, 1957, p. 302).

Donor offspring have also been called child, children, babies, people conceived through DI, a donated child, the AID child (artificial insemination by donor), custom-made child, and turkey-baster babies. (Daniels and Haimes, 1998, p. 54).

> The labeling of such people as 'babies' can suggest that they are to be seen as merely the end-product of DI, whereas labeling them 'children', 'offspring', 'adults', 'people' can suggest that they have lives and biographies with the potential to extend beyond their origins in DI. (Daniels and Haimes, 1998, p. 54)

"Donor insemination" (DI) originally was called "artificial insemination by donor" (AID). After the acronym AIDS (auto-immune disease) came into wide use, and due to disagreement with the term "artificial," AID became known as DI or donor insemination.

The terminology, a reflection of the understanding of the nature of the relationships, has been unclear and controversial. Baran and Pannor (1993), in their classic book on donor insemination, were instrumental in defining the terminology in the field (pp. 3-4). They call the sperm donor the "donor father" or "genetic father," and they call the person conceived from DI the "donor offspring." Commonly, the term "social father" is used for the father who raises the child. He is also the "legal father." "Donor conception", or DC, refers to conception using donor sperm or eggs.

Other terminology for "donor offspring" is sometimes used. Cordray (1999/2000, p. 3) states that he prefers to be called a "DI adoptee." His reasoning is that the term "insemination" raises images of animal insemination, which is where the procedure started. Also, the donor situation is similar to an adoptive situation, where a child is raised by a non-biological parent and is considered the legal child of that person.

In DI, traditionally, there is one biological parent (the mother) and one "adoptive" parent (the social father). There are, of course, variations on the configuration of the families, e.g., single mothers or lesbian couples.

In fact, some of the psychological components are the same in both adoption and DI situations, for example, identity issues and "genealogical bewilderment."

> In 1952, Wellisch coined the phrase "genealogical bewilderment," which refers to no knowledge, or uncertain knowledge, of at least one biological parent. He found that the resulting state of confusion and uncertainty undermines the child's security and affects his mental health, meaning that he has no stable concept of himself and his status. (Noble, 1987, p. 292)

I understand this desire to find more fitting terminology, but I decided to stay with the more common terminology of "donor offspring" for this study.

Putting the definitions all together then, the meaning of the thesis question "What is the experience of confronting the reality of being a donor offspring?" is: What is the resulting knowledge (thoughts, feelings, sensations, behavior, interactions) of actively pursuing the meaning of unmasking the denial of being a person conceived through donor insemination?

I ask the co-researchers in this study to describe their personal experiences and inner knowledge as a result of actively confronting the reality of being a donor offspring. Through phenomenological reduction, I look for common themes in the experience of confronting the reality of being a donor offspring.

CHAPTER III
REVIEW OF LITERATURE

In this chapter, I review the literature on the psychology of donor offspring and in particular, look for previous research related to donor offspring confronting the reality of this situation. The focus is on seeking the meaning of the experience of being an offspring of donor insemination. I did an extensive review of the literature including research results, journal articles, medical resources, media reports, and personal accounts in books and magazine articles. The list of resources related to donor insemination and donor offspring which I find useful to my interests in the field are included in the resource section at the back of this report (References and Appendix A).

I found a vast amount of printed material related to donor insemination available. Research has been done from the point of view of all of the participants in the DI realm: offspring, parents, donors, physicians, and social workers and other health practitioners. In this chapter, I review the research resources describing the experience of the offspring themselves.

I did not include all of the resources I discovered in Appendix A. There are also more resources related to specific populations using donor insemination, e.g., single mothers and lesbian couples. I included these resources only if they were relevant to the experience of the offspring confronting the reality of the situation. Research on the experience of these more specific populations is important but is not the focus of this particular study.

I also did not include all of the resources available related to the Christian perspective of donor insemination, specific to other cultures, payment issues, and other assisted reproductive techniques, e.g. egg and embryo donation, in vitro fertilization (IVF), gamete intrafallopian transfer (GIFT), and zygote intrafallopian transfer (ZIFT). Again, I only included these perspectives if I felt they were specifically related to the experience of donor offspring.

In the media resources, there are a lot of articles about recent lawsuits pertaining to paternity and custody issues and the rights to use of gametes which I also did not include. I did include information about the ethics, policy, and regulation issues related to donor insemination.

I reviewed the literature without limits on the year it was published. My literature search originally covered up to the year 2000, and has since been updated. Although human donor insemination was first documented in 1884 in western culture, the literature does not start until 1951 and only then sporadically. There is a history of secrecy in the field which is apparent in the lack of early literature. I find the historical view important and therefore did not limit the data search as to when it was written. It will be important for the reader to pay attention to the timing of the different resources, as this shows the evolution of the practice of donor insemination.

There has been another impediment in studying the experience of donor offspring. Due to the belief system that secrecy was best, the majority of donor offspring do not know their status as a donor offspring. They do not know that their social father is not also their biological father. If the people involved do not know that they are part of the population, their experience as part of that population can not be studied.

Thus, the research on the perspective from the donor offspring has been very limited. It has only come into view in about the last twenty years. More and more, the policy of secrecy in donor insemination is being questioned. I have included resources related to secrecy in the reference section.

Donor insemination is done around the world. Technically, it is a simple procedure, and can be performed anywhere. There is a trend towards greater disclosure and concern about ethical issues. I have included some resources from around the world relevant to the experience of the offspring.

I have chosen to list some resources from more public or popular literature which are less research based. My study is about hearing the voice of the donor offspring. This has often occurred in the popular literature, rather than in scientific studies. Since my research is qualitative and experientially based, I find that these resources are relevant to mention, and actually vitally relevant to the research at hand. They are personal stories about the experiences of donor offspring from their perspective.

My next task was to narrow the focus of available information and position my study within the existing research. I used two criteria when selecting resources to review to position my research: (1) that it be research based, and (2) that the information was from the voice of the offspring themselves. I found two resources which strictly met these criteria, Geithner (1988) and Turner (1999). I describe these references, and then others in less detail. I explain how my research fits in or is related to these studies

Geithner (1988) was the first to interview adult donor offspring about their experiences for research purposes. She performed an exploratory/ descriptive analysis focusing on secrecy. She interviewed seven offspring, ranging in age from 16 to 44. They found out their identity as donor offspring between 11 and 35 years old. She interviewed people in person or over the phone, and had a long list of questions she asked them about themselves, their families, and their feelings related to secrecy, identity, and relationships. The conclusions were that those interviewed were upset about the way they learned they were DI offspring. They felt that their social father was distant. They wanted more information about their donor father, at least medical information. They felt that donor offspring should be told the truth of their origins prior to the age of 18. Recommendations included keeping medical records on sperm donors, educating and counseling DI parents about the implications of donor insemination, and advising them to tell the offspring of their origins.

Turner (1999) focused on the identity experiences of adult donor offspring. She did a qualitative analysis using Interpretative Phenomenological Analysis. She recruited sixteen donor offspring internationally. Their ages ranged from 26 to 55. Research participants completed a questionnaire in writing which consisted of 27 questions relating to identity experiences and relationships. The themes expressed by the donor offspring were: life as a lie/mistrust, withholding information and the effects on the family/parental marital dynamics, the need to know/making genetic connections, searching for the donor, and talking—the need for significant others. Her research concludes that there may be psychological implications for therapy based on issues of trust, self-esteem, insecurity in family relationships, a need to talk, and being undervalued socially.

My research continues in this vein. It is also a qualitative type of research, a phenomenological analysis. I focused on the older adult offspring who knew of their origins. Their ages ranged from 39 to 57. They found out about their status as a donor offspring between the ages of 18 and 47. I conducted interviews with donor offspring in person or over the phone. The main difference with my research is that after a few initial bibliographic specific questions, the interview became open-ended. This allowed for whatever was important in the experience of the person to become a part of the research. The themes presented by the research participants validated the themes from Geithner's and Turner's research, but new themes were presented as well.

At the time of this research, I was not able to find any other original research projects from the voice of the donor offspring. O'Brien (1996) did her senior honors thesis on <u>Artificial Insemination by Donor: The Voice of the Unborn Child</u>. Her thesis is a literature review. She focuses on the history of AID, secrecy, genetic versus social parenting, morals, and negligence in the system of DI. She concludes that morals need to be considered before using a donor in procreation. The child has a right to know his or her identity. The donor is by nature connected to the child. She stresses the importance of protecting the well being of the child, including legal rights, the right to medical information and the need for an accepting attitude from society.

Cordray (1999/2000) conducted an informal survey of 36 "DI adoptees", his terminology for donor offspring. Ages ranged from 12 to 56. They were from the United States, Australia, United Kingdom, and Canada. He asked specific questions related to secrecy, doubt about paternity, relationships, and rights to know medical information and identity of donor. The conclusions from this group of DI adoptees is that they support disclosure between the ages of 5 and 10 years old and that they feel information about their genetic history and the identity of the donor is their right.

Baran and Pannor (1993) conducted interviews with donor offspring, husbands (some infertile and some with vasectomies) and wives in donor insemination families, lesbian women, single women, and donors. The donor offspring ranged in age between 16 and 68 years of age. Their goal was an exploratory analysis of the emotional and psychological effects of donor insemination on all of the parties involved. They offer recommendations for each group of people, including:

The donor offspring:

1 Must be accepted as having two genetic parents who are important to him; they contribute to his identity and self-concept. They connect him to his biological and historical past and provide him with information that is vital to his health and well-being.

2 Has a right to know, at an appropriate age, of his DI conception.

3 Has a right to know the identity of the donor father and his medical, social, and familial information.

4 Has a right to meet his donor father if he wishes to have personal contact. (Baran and Pannor, 1993, p. 168)

I was unable to find a copy of Achilles (1987) dissertation The Social Meaning of Biological Ties: A Study of Participants in Artificial Insemination by Donor. This may possibly contain interviews with donor offspring about their experiences.

Research which contained information about the adjustment of children from the point of view of the parents or clinicians include: Chan, Raboy, and Patterson (1998), Golombok, Murray, Brinsden, and Abdalla (1999), Kovacs, Mushin, Kane, Baker (1993), and Leeton, Backwell (1982).

More general literature research regarding the welfare of donor offspring includes: Berger (1982), Blyth, Crawshaw, Speirs (1998), Daniels, Haimes (1998), NZPA (2000), Sokoloff (1987), Stotland (1990), and Verny (1994).

Resources where donor offspring are directly quoted, but are not research based, include: Blyth, Crawshaw, Speirs (1998), Botsford (2000), Briggs (1997), Brown (1994), Burleigh (1999), Children of Sperm Donors (1998), Cobb (1992), Donor Conception Support Group of Australia (1997), Franz (2000), Kinross (1992), Landsberg (2000), Norton (2000), Orenstein (1995), Rubin (1995), Topp (1993), and White (1998).

CHAPTER IV
PHENOMENOLOGICAL RESEARCH MODEL

In this chapter, I explain the history of phenomenological philosophy, psychology, and research. The steps of the phenomenological research process are described. This is the model used for this research study.

The intent of phenomenology is the discovery of meaning in human experience. Understanding the history and philosophy of phenomenology is helpful in understanding its importance for research. Moustakas (1994, p. 26) describes some of the roots of phenomenology:

> For Hegel, phenomenology referred to knowledge as it appears to consciousness, the science of describing what one perceives, senses, and knows in one's immediate awareness and experience...What appears in consciousness is the phenomenon. The word *phenomenon* comes from the Greek *phaenesthai*, to flare up, to show itself, to appear. Constructed from *phaino,* phenomenon means to bring to light, to place in brightness, to show itself in itself, the totality of what lies before us in the light of day.

> Valle (1998, p. 5) aptly describes Husserl's original ideas about phenomenology:
> As the originator of philosophical phenomenology, Husserl articulated the central insight that consciousness is intentional, that is, that human consciousness is always and essentially oriented toward a world of emergent meaning...Experiences are constituted by consciousness and thus could be rigorously and systematically studied on the basis of their appearances to consciousness-that is, their phenomenal nature.

Besides being a philosophy, phenomenology is a type of psychological practice and a research method. Adrian van Kaam, founder of the doctoral psychology department at Duquesne University, was fundamental in founding psychology as a human science. From there, phenomenological psychology has continued to develop. Many people have contributed to the phenomenological paradigm, including Husserl, Kant, Hegel, Descartes, Sartre, and Buber.

> Our existential-phenomenological psychology is continuously in evolution. In our attempts to deepen our understanding of the meaning of human existence, we are constantly questioning our presuppositions and forever challenging our tendencies to reach premature closure. Thus, while we are reasonably certain of our overall direction and the goals towards which we are striving, we want to remain open to change; we seek to deliberately avoid any dogmatic stance...To study man as a human being, rather than as a human organism or as a human machine, has meant that we are now challenged by the problem of capturing the full depth and diversity of human living. Our only problem, and it is a truly monumental one, is that of finding those methodological and conceptual tools that will enable us to do justice to the phenomena that we seek to understand. (Giorgi, Fischer, & Von Eckartsberg 1971, vi)

Qualitative research, in general, seeks to find understanding of human experience from the person's own frame of reference. Cook (1979, p. 10) describes the qualitative paradigm as "grounded, discovery-oriented, exploratory, expansionist, descriptive, and inductive."

Phenomenological research is one type of qualitative research. Phenomenological research seeks to find meaning in people's experience. "In accordance with phenomenological principles, scientific investigation is valid when the knowledge sought is arrived at through descriptions that make possible an understanding of the meanings and essences of experience" (Moustakas, 1994, p. 84). In this research study, I interview donor offspring in order for them to describe their experience of confronting the reality of being a donor offspring.

Karlsson describes the differences between phenomenological and traditional psychological approaches to research: qualitative v. quantitative, descriptive v. explanatory, meaning v. facts, openness v. hypothesis testing, the "inside" v. the "outside" perspective, hermeneutical ("aims at deepening our understanding of phenomena") v. technical interest, life-world studies v. laboratory set-ups, and consciousness as intentionality v. consciousness as something "thing-like" (1993, pp. 13-19).

Traditional quantitative research, and qualitative research, such as phenomenological, both have their place in the world and in the field of psychology. Speaking of qualitative research, Patton states: "There is indeed a viable alternative to the dominant natural science model, an alternative that not only employs different methods but also asks different questions" (1975, p. 17). The type of research method that is appropriate depends on the questions asked, and the intention and meaning sought in the research. In studying the experience of confronting the reality of being a donor offspring, a qualitative approach is appropriate to study individual experience.

Phenomenological research involves the following steps: epoche, phenomenological reduction (including bracketing, horizonalizing, clustering into themes, and textural description), imaginative variation, and synthesis. I use these steps in the study of donor offspring's experience. They are described in the following text.

EPOCHE

Epoche is a Greek word meaning to stay away from or abstain. In the context of phenomenological research, epoche means to set aside our judgments and biases. We let go of our preconceived ideas in order to allow "things, events, and people to enter anew into consciousness, and to look and see them again, as if for the first time" (Moustakas, 1994, p. 85). We clear our minds and become open, in order to allow new awareness, feelings, and understanding of our experience. As Moustakas states, "it is a way of genuine looking that precedes reflectiveness, the making of judgments, or reaching conclusions" (1994, p. 86).

The purpose of epoche is to be able to experience the true nature of something and get to its essential meaning. It requires full concentration, being in the here and now with the experience. "I return to the original nature of my conscious experience" (Moustakas, 1994, p. 87). In getting to our own individual consciousness, we must set aside thoughts of others' perceptions or judgments, as well. If preconceived notions enter our consciousness, we acknowledge them, wait for them to clear, so that we can view our experience with clarity and new meaning.

Epoche offers a resource, a process for potential renewal. Approached with dedication and determination, the process can make a difference in what and how we see, hear, and/or view things. Practiced wisely, realistically, and with determination to let go of our prejudices, I believe that the actual nature and essence of things will be disclosed more fully, will reveal themselves to us and enable us to find a clearing and light to knowledge and truth. (Moustakas, 1994, p. 90).

PHENOMENOLOGICAL REDUCTION

The next stage of phenomenological research is phenomenological reduction. This step involves describing the experience. We look and describe, look again and describe, and so on. We look at the phenomenon externally, in our internal consciousness, and the relationship between the phenomenon and the self. We perceive the experience from different angles and describe it. The phenomenon is viewed in its pure state with the intention of uncovering its essential meaning.

Bracketing

The first stage of phenomenological reduction is bracketing. In bracketing, the phenomenon being researched is placed in brackets, that is the focus is solely on the particular experience being studied. Anything unrelated is set aside.

The experiencing person turns inward and reflects. Whatever perceptions come forth in consciousness are attended to. The focus is on the center of the experience, viewing it just as it appears. After looking and looking again, a more reflective process evolves.

> The whole process of reducing toward what is texturally meaningful and essential in its phenomenal and experiential components depends on competent and clear reflectiveness, on an ability to attend, recognize, and describe with clarity. Reflection becomes more exact and fuller with continuing attention and perception, with continued looking, with the adding of new perspectives. Reflection becomes more exact through corrections that more completely and accurately present what appears before us. Things become clearer as they are considered again and again. (Moustakas, 1994, p. 93)

Horizonalization

One of the steps of phenomenological reduction is horizonalization. We seek to find the essence and meaning of what we are viewing. At this stage, we describe the constituents of the essential bracketed phenomenon.

Each phenomenon, or description of the experience, initially has equal value.

> Horizons are unlimited. We can never exhaust completely our experience of things no matter how many times we reconsider them or view them. A new horizon arises each time that one recedes. It is a never-ending process and, though we may reach a stopping point and discontinue our perception of something, the possibility for discovery is unlimited. (Moustakas, 1994, p. 95)

By continuing to reflect on the experience, new horizons become apparent. Qualities are recognized and we describe the horizons of the phenomenon as the invariant constituents of the research.

<u>Clustering the Horizons into Themes</u>

The next step in the phenomenological reduction is looking for themes in the descriptions of the horizons. Statements irrelevant to the topic and question as well as those that are repetitive or overlapping are deleted. The remaining essential constituents are sorted into themes. Themes may relate to relationship to self or others, relationship to spirituality, feelings, bodily reactions, pain, memories, concerns or difficulties, personal meanings attached to things, decisions, life changes, integration of new aspects of the authentic self or identity, alteration of personal values, incorporating new meanings, visions or fantasies, influence of time or space, or internal or external barriers to the experience.

<u>Organizing the Horizons and Themes Into a Coherent Textural Description</u>

The final stage of the phenomenological reduction is completing a complete textural description of the discovered horizons and themes. The essential constituents of the experience are described fully. The phenomenological reduction enables "an uncovering of the nature and meaning of experience, bringing the experiencing person to a self-knowledge and a knowledge of the phenomenon" (Moustakas, 1994, p. 97).

IMAGINATIVE VARIATION

The next step in phenomenological research is imaginative variation. The goal of imaginative variation is to find the pure essence of the experience. We describe the essential structures of the phenomenon, and by permitting all possibilities to enter our consciousness, we uncover the essences of the experience being studied. The goal is finding the meaning in the experience.

The steps of imaginative variation are:

1 Systematic varying of the possible structural meanings that under lie the textural meanings;

2 Recognizing the underlying themes or contexts that account for the emergence of the phenomenon;

3 Considering the universal structures that precipitate feelings and thoughts with reference to the phenomenon, such as the structure of time, space, bodily concerns, materiality, causality, relation to self, or relation to others;

4 Searching for exemplifications that vividly illustrate the invariant structural themes and facilitate the development of a structural description of the phenomenon. (Moustakas, 1994, p. 99)

Imaginative variation allows us to find structural themes from the textural descriptions that we developed in the phenomenological reduction stage.

SYNTHESIS OF MEANINGS AND ESSENCES

The last step of phenomenological research is developing a statement about the essence of the phenomenon studied as a whole. Essence is that which is common or universal to the experience. Without the qualities of its essence, the phenomenon would not be what it is.

Phenomenological research studies the essence of a phenomenon at a particular place and time. Experience is infinite, so the essences of an experience are never totally derived. The way is always open for further explorations into an experience.

The synthesis then is the integration of the textural and structural descriptions and themes from the previous stages of the phenomenological research. New knowledge and meaning is gained from the state of pure consciousness about a particular segment of human experience.

By using the qualitative phenomenological research method, I have discovered themes and the essence of the experience of confronting the reality of being a donor offspring.

CHAPTER V
METHODS AND PROCEDURES

The first step in qualitative research methodology is "discovering a topic and question rooted in autobiographical meanings and values, as well as involving social meanings and significance." (Moustakas, 1994, p. 103). My topic is "What is the experience of confronting the reality of being a donor offspring?"

The next stage in phenomenological research is to develop criteria for the co-researchers and the method of locating them. My co-researchers are donor offspring. A further criteria is that they have actively been involved in a process of confronting the reality of being a donor offspring. What does this mean? By confronting the reality, I mean that they have immersed themselves in the process of discovering what being a donor offspring means to them in their lives—to them personally, their perceptions of identity, and in relation to others in their lives. It might involve reaching out to others, seeking others to talk to and process being a donor offspring. It could involve calling others, searching the internet, or in some way reaching out to find other people who are donor offspring, sharing their experience with others, seeking support, or breaking the code of secrecy. It could involve accessing DI support groups, speaking out in the media, or participating in research projects related to donor insemination. The important piece is that they have been in the process of confronting what being a donor offspring means to them.

Due to the secrecy surrounding donor insemination, a lot of people do not know their status as a donor offspring or for any number of reasons, choose to maintain a level of secrecy and do not seek others or share their stories with others. The donor offspring in this study are those who have actively been involved in a discovery process of what being a donor offspring means to them in their lives.

One last criteria for the co-researchers in this research study is an age factor. Most studies of the effects of donor insemination on the offspring involve interviews with the parents of young children. This is important, but I feel that more information needs to be obtained from offspring who are older and have more experience with what donor insemination means in their lives. Due to the limited number of people available to participate in this study, I did not set a firm age requirement. I focused on the older end of the age range of potential participants. My co-researchers' ages range from 39 to 57.

Through my own personal discovery process in being a donor offspring, I have developed a network of acquaintances in the field. They, in turn, have larger networks of contacts of people involved in donor insemination. I contacted my network of acquaintances, via phone and e-mail, explained my research project, and asked them for referrals of those people who met the criteria for co-researchers.

Next, I contacted possible co-researchers, via phone, e-mail, or mail, explained the research project and requirements for participation, and asked if they were willing to participate in the study. If they agreed to participate, I sent them, via mail or e-mail, an Instructions to Research Participants sheet (see Appendix C) and a Participation Release Agreement (see Appendix D). Once I received their signed agreement form, I contacted the co-researcher, via phone or e-mail, to arrange a time for the research interview. We selected a time when we both had one to two hours of uninterrupted, private time available.

As much as possible, I conducted the interviews in person. I offered to co-researchers to meet in my home or their home, whichever was more comfortable for them. I was able to interview two co-researchers face-to-face, one in my home and one in her home. Due to the geographical dispersion of co-researchers who met the criteria for this study, six of the interviews were done over the phone. Whether the interview was done in person or over the phone, I recorded the interview with an audio tape recorder in order to be able to transcribe the interview.

I developed guiding questions for my interviews with co-researchers (see Appendix F). The goal of the interviews was to create an environment where the co-researchers felt comfortable sharing their feelings, thoughts, and actions related to their experience of confronting the reality of being a donor offspring. I began the interview with an epoche period for myself and the co-researcher. I set aside my preconceived notions about the experience of confronting the reality of being a donor offspring, relaxed, and focused on the co-researcher and the guiding questions. I asked the co-researchers to think about times when being a donor offspring was central to their experiencing, e.g. finding out about it, talking to others about it, thinking about it, taking action on it, or other times when being a donor offspring was significant for them in their lives. I asked them to describe their feelings, their thoughts, and their actions while actively processing being a donor offspring.

The research participants were all open with their feelings about confronting the reality of being a donor offspring. They shared honestly about their feelings and reactions to this experience. During the interview, some people experienced a high level of emotion, and were teary off and on throughout the interview. At some point during the interview, everyone said they were done or that was all they could think of related to confronting being a donor offspring. As we sat in respectful silence, other things would then arise for them, and the interview would continue. The interviews lasted from twenty minutes to 1-1/2 hours, most of them toward the longer end of this range. The interviews ended when people had exhausted what was relevant for them in confronting the reality of being a donor offspring.

At the conclusion of the interview, I offered to co-researchers to contact me, via phone or e-mail, if other feelings or thoughts became relevant to them in relation to confronting the reality of being a donor offspring. I also reminded them that I may possibly need to contact them one more time to clarify information from our initial interview.

Some of the co-researchers expressed a desire to have their real names used in the research. One donor offspring wrote on the original Participation Release Agreement form, "OK to make my info public!! OK to use my name! NOT A SECRET!!" As a result of these expressed desires to have their real names used in the research, I explored the issue of confidentiality with my thesis advisor. We looked in the Ethical Principles of Psychologists and Code of Conduct (American Psychological Association, 1992, p. 11). Guidelines for ethics in research are that limitations to confidentiality must be done with written informed consent from the participant. As a result, I sent a new release agreement letter to participants (see Appendix E). In the letter, it explains the desire of some participants to use their real names, the ethical standards for disclosure, and the proposed use of information from the research study. Co-researchers returned the letters with their written consent for how they wish to be addressed in the publication of this research data.

I interviewed eight co-researchers for this study. Four were male and four were female. Five were conceived using donor insemination in the United States, and three were conceived in the United Kingdom. The age of being informed about being a donor offspring ranged from 18 to 47. More information about the circumstances of being told about DI and sibling relationships is found in Appendix G.

The next stage in this phenomenological study was to transcribe the interviews. From there, I analyzed the interview data to determine the themes and develop textural and structural descriptions, and a synthesis of textural and structural meanings and essences (see Chapter VI). I used the phenomenological research model to derive the meaning from the interviews with co-researchers who confront the reality of being a donor offspring.

CHAPTER VI
THE EXPERIENCES OF DONOR OFFSPRING

HANDLING AND PRESENTATION OF DATA
PHENOMENOLOGICAL REDUCTION

After completing the interviews and transcribing them, I analyzed the data using a phenomenological method of analysis. I performed the phenomenological reduction. First I bracketed the information from the open-ended interviews, setting aside anything which did not fit into the research question of "What is the experience of confronting the reality of being a donor offspring?" Then I used horizonalization by giving each phenomenon (description of the experience) within the topic equal value. From this, I clustered the horizons into 15 themes.

Themes

The themes presented in these research interviews are:
1. Regret, anger, and feeling of injustice regarding secrecy of the reality of being a donor offspring
2. Feeling different, discomfort telling others due to lack of understanding by others of the donor offspring's experience
3. Doubt about paternity, feeling of not fitting in family (before knowing about being a donor offspring)
4. Identity confusion
5. Search for the sperm donor, need for ancestral connection
6. Search for half-siblings, feeling a connection with them
7. Concern about next generation and inherited medical conditions
8. Feeling alone as a donor offspring, having a need for contact with others and support
9. Finding support and similar experiences in adoption groups
10. Need to seek out information about donor insemination

11. Positive feelings: being special, interesting, wanted, grateful to be alive
12. Negative thoughts and feelings: troubled, angry, injustice, loss, nonexistence, split feelings
13. Wanting to normalize being a donor offspring, accepting the reality
14. Developed beliefs that knowledge of genetic and medical history are a birthright
15. Becoming an activist, finding a sense of purpose, duty to speak up.

Following is a description of each theme derived from the interviews with donor offspring, followed by quotes from individual co-researchers. I used the co-researchers statements verbatim, as much as possible, changing wording without changing the meaning only to put the statements in appropriate context for the reader. At times I will clarify in parenthesis who the co-researcher is referring to.

1. <u>Regret, anger, and feeling of injustice regarding secrecy of the reality of being a donor offspring</u>

Co-researchers expressed many strong feelings against secrecy. They uniformly felt that it was best to know from an early age that they were donor offspring. When only some of the children in the family were told about being donor offspring, there was an insistence to tell the others as well. Alliances and distance developed in families because of keeping the secret.

I really regret that he (father) hadn't been able to tell the secret at an early age. He never did tell me.

The other thing I felt was a whole lot of sadness, mainly for having been deprived of being able to have discussed it (DI) with my father. I think I would have really enjoyed talking about the whole thing with him. My hunch is we would have been able to talk and have some good conversations with him and not rejected him, which I think is probably what all fathers fear, that they're going to be rejected by these offspring who are not biologically theirs. But we loved him. He was our father.

My father, I never had the feeling he liked me very much. When I look back on it, after I knew about the donor insemination, it made sense, because I don't think he really felt like he was my father. I think he felt remote from me because of that, and to a certain extent, resented me, because of that. And that is painful. And I always felt guilty because I didn't love him more. It's paradoxical, he is my father, and that's just a fact, but it's as though he didn't feel as though he was. And that's really sad, because it's so unnecessary. I would have been delighted had he felt like more my father.

He (a clinic doctor) said something that just really, really hurt hard. It was that he felt it was very important to never tell the child. That made me extremely angry. Everything he was saying just irritated me.

This dynamic in families, and artificial insemination is part of it, that it's okay to lie. And so the doctor is in on the lie, the nurse or secretary is in on the lie, the parents are in on the lie, the donor is probably in on the lie. It's a lie. It's stealing. It's injustice, unfairness. We've been robbed. I had a sense of unfairness to start with from our family. I mean the whole thing was the loyalty to the lie. The devotion to this dishonesty was enormous. It's above everything. The whole thing is not a healthy dynamic.

I would love to know anything about myself. I hate not knowing anything. I think secrets are awful. I think they're lethal.

I think it's better not to (keep it secret). I think it's better to, just like a child who is adopted, you raise just knowing you were adopted. Then it's not an issue.

Certainly in my experience, a child is going to, not that you necessarily know, but the parents know, and it's going to affect them and their interaction, and the father's going to know. And if you aren't talking about it, then why aren't you talking about it? Well, because you think it's a problem. And if you think it's a problem, then it's affecting the family. It's there in your mind, and it's there bunging up communication, and being a barrier to closeness in the family. A secret is definitely a barrier to closeness in the family. What I think is that secrecy, the people who advocate secrecy, who are advocating lying and deception, should have to justify their position.

When I was forty eight, I insisted on telling my other siblings about it.

When I saw our father, I wanted to discuss the artificial insemination with him, but I hadn't yet told my siblings. In other words, I felt I should keep the secret for our mother. But I sort of chafed under it. I then knew about the artificial insemination, and he didn't know I knew about it.

2. Feeling different, discomfort telling others due to lack of understanding by others of their experience

Not everyone spoke about the theme of telling others that they are donor offspring. Those who did, felt a sense that others did not understand why it was important to them, unless they were offspring or adoptees themselves. There was a sense of being different from other people. As a result, they were selective about who they told.

I tried telling my closest friends, and it didn't really work, because you find out that everybody has fertility issues. I realized that I just had to stay away from it. So I told a few people, and that was that. I never told anyone else. Maybe because I felt different. And most people basically said, "What's the big deal?" It is a big deal. Unless you're an adopted person, you don't know what it feels like. It's okay. Everyone that I'm close to is supportive.

There is a difference between myself and other people. Some other people, who don't necessarily understand what it's like to be the offspring of a donor, that there's something there that they don't know about, that they have never experienced.

I shared that part of my history with my soon-to-be husband. It was just that this is where I come from. He was very open and understanding, and was very accepting, so it wasn't a big deal. I wanted to make sure that if he was going to stay with me and we were going to be a couple, that he knew. When I had my daughter, I started talking to her, my biological daughter. I chose not to tell anybody else, all the way up until about a year and a half ago.

Because I had kept it secret for quite a long time, or it just wasn't talked about, that told me that there was part of me that had some feelings about it, some discomfort perhaps, in sharing it with people. I wouldn't use as strong a word as shame, but discomfort probably. I wrote out on the internet, e-mails to people, to infertility networks, in a fairly anonymous way. I think I became more bold because everyone shared so much of themselves with me. So I started being more open, too.

This is not anything that people wanted to talk about, right? I guess I wasn't surprised how people react when you tell them, because it happened over and over again when I would tell people.

3. Doubt about paternity, feeling of not fitting in family (before knowing about being a donor offspring)

Half of the co-researchers sensed that their fathers were not their biological fathers, that they were adopted. or that something was different in their families. They had strong feelings about this and their stories are quite striking.

There was this overwhelming resurgence of feelings of doubt about my paternity. And so I was thinking I wonder if there is a slight possibility that my dad wasn't really my father. When I was talking with my mother, there was this look on her face. It made me realize I touched on some kind of a nerve from the inheritance business. When I was five I had asked my mother if I was adopted, and so even at that age I was aware that I wasn't like my dad. I think I was starting to fantasize that my mother had had an affair. I didn't look like my dad or feel any kind of kinship with him. There were whole parts of my personality that were totally different from both of my parents that must have come from my donor. Well, it was very confusing. I felt like a stranger in my own family. I felt so totally alienated, or alone, in my family, even though I think that the family dynamics were fairly strong. We were a relatively close family.

Between my father and me, we had absolutely nothing physical in common. He was five feet one, and weighed about 120 pounds, and I was six feet tall and 170. I was blonde hair and light complected. He was dark hair with dark complexion. I wondered all the time. I questioned my mom if I was adopted, oh, when I was about 9, 10, 11 years old. She said she gave birth to me. She was telling half the truth. That generally will squelch any further curiosity, but I would always look at my father and try to find something in common. I could never find anything.

My parents were very, very—and probably that was part of protecting the secret, but they were very withdrawn. They're not outgoing people, and certainly I'm very outgoing. I could never understand. "Where does that come from?" I would say. "Where did I come from?" At one point, I had asked the question to my parents, when I was 29.

I probably just always had a feeling that something was different. I can remember a scene when I was about 10, and I just thought maybe I was adopted. And I can remember sitting in seventh grade and they put me beside a girl that was born at the same hospital the same day, and to me she's a spitting image of my mother. And I always used to think that we had been switched.

I had kind of guessed that something was not right between me and my father, and that there was something strange in the relationship between my mother and my father that I couldn't really fathom. And I was sitting in the kitchen one day talking to my mother and the subject of my relationship with my father came up as it did quite often. And I just kind of knew, and I just thought I'm going to ask now whether he is actually my father, because I had sensed that he wasn't. And so I asked my mother, and at first she denied it. But I just got very angry with her and ended up shouting at her and saying that "you ought to tell me. It's my right to know." And so she did.

4. Identity confusion

Identity issues were fundamental for these donor offspring, and were a big focus in the interviews. Even before knowing that they were donor offspring, they had confusion about why they were different from their families in some ways. After they found out their status as a donor offspring, there was a need to incorporate this as a part of who they were. There was confusion and wondering about which parts of them came from the sperm donor. This was sometimes triggered when people asked questions about who they look like or who their children look like. Knowing they were donor offspring helped clarify the incongruities of their characteristics within their families. Accepting themselves as donor offspring was a part of accepting their identity, or who they were as a person.

Even though I had some similarities with my mother, it seemed like a greater part of me just came out of the blue.

I was feeling very confused. It's just not knowing what your roots are.

When my mother told me (about DI), I had to go through a major readjustment of my self-concept, self-image.

What is this donor insemination stuff about? I thought that I was really weird. I said, "Who am I?" I was very confused. Who is this guy who donated? Right handed? Left handed? What are his interests? I mean, half of me—I became an enigma, a mystery.

Certainly that (DI) was the revelation, in a sense, which explained everything—why I'm so very different. I'm very different than my parents. And I see things differently, very differently. I didn't understand that. I don't really look like my mother. I must look like my donor. It's really hard not knowing my history, my genealogy.

I still feel like there's a line drawn down the half of me, and I know one half, and the other half is just this other person that I can only identify that she's left handed, she talks too much, she's outgoing, all these little idiosyncrasies that are totally different than the rest of the family.

People will ask things about, "Do your kids look like somebody?" That's when I start thinking about it, because I start wondering who this man is, and what he looks like, and who he is.

I went to see my therapist for the first time. I was unbelievably surprised when the very first thing I said to her as I sat down was "I think I ought to tell you, before we get started, I'm a donor offspring." I explained to her what it meant. I had no idea that it was so central to who I was. I had no idea of the importance it had for me. The fact that I couldn't be me without telling her that first. It was a turning point in a sense. In fact, the process of therapy was part of the discovery about exactly what it had meant to me, and what effects it had on me.

I don't think it has affected my identity in some senses. I don't think it changes the core. I am who I am. But it changes my identity in that I am part of the family who I grew up with, but I've also inherited some characteristics and genetics that were connected to a very different kind of family. I always had a sense that I was slightly different. Now I realized that I am actually half Jewish, and half from Russia. That totally makes sense to me. It totally explains a lot of things to me. It explains my emotional expressiveness. And I enjoy really talking about things, in great depth. You're going around with a lot of hunches about who you are. I think when one doesn't know, one seeks an explanation for the way one is sometimes. It's because you don't know—you don't know whether that might be an inherited characteristic, or if you've inherited temperament from somebody else, or why you've become particularly interested in that. I used to joke that I thought I was probably Jewish. I always had a very natural way with Jewish people. I was always easily accepted into that kind of community. It became kind of special after I found out, because they always acknowledge their own. So I guess they must have thought I looked Jewish. There was some recognition there, I think, at some subliminal level, which is very interesting to me.

My brother and I, who was there, and my mom, all of us were looking at each other. He and I were particularly looking at each other, and looking at my mom, and trying to figure out—you know, looking at lengths of fingers, and looking at facial characteristics, and trying to figure out what parts of us belong to this strange new person (sperm donor) who'd kind of come into our lives. Of course, you can't isolate noses, or mouths, or ears, or whatever, because half of us come from our mother genetically. So we weren't able to do that. But anyway, it was really kind of an amazing time.

An identity issue, that was the other thing that I'm very aware of. I've always been pretty comfortable with who I am, and the different facets of who I am. But, of course, that means then accepting the fact that I am the offspring of an unknown donor…As I got closer to 50, I personally felt an increasing sense of comfort as to who I am, and embracing all the parts, which includes that part, and then confronting the thoughts about it, and realizing that that's okay. I mean, so what if I came from a turkey baster, or whatever. I'm still me and I'm still happy with who I am.

For me, it (being a donor offspring) is a big deal. It is a part of who

I am. There's a certain part of me, my identity, that feels like I do have some belonging to that other person (donor) who made me, in some way. I feel as if I would like to know who that person is. I'm just curious, what their life has been like, what their interests are, whether they have some similar characteristics as I do, which is possible, and maybe likely even—not so much how I look, but more like what internally goes on inside me and how that relates to this other person whose sperm I might come from. To be a person who is born and conceived from a donor, other than the parent, needs to be raised with that knowledge and to accept that and know thyself right from the beginning.

What it (DI) does is call into question basic ideas about identity, what identity is, and who we are. It is pretty interesting to try to figure out what the meaning of this thing is. When you split off the two functions of father, if you like, the biological function and the social function, then it does throw into relief the differences between them, and it throws into relief the different components of our selves.

At the time we were told, I assumed that we did not have the same donor father, and that's how we were accepting things for many years. We don't look that alike, and so that was how it was, until we found out yes indeed through DNA testing we are whole siblings, which is very exciting.

5. Search for the sperm donor, need for ancestral connection

Experiencing a desire for ancestral connection was an important theme for co-researchers. They searched for their sperm donors. Frustration was intensely felt, in not knowing how to seek out their donors, and uncertainty about finding them. The fear of rejection delayed the search. With limited information, people fantasized or leaped to conclusions, because they had such a strong need for answers as to who their donor was.

I immediately started searching, or started trying to figure out who the guy was. That became a bit obsessive, and so the impact of that was pretty strong, because it was so frustrating trying to find out any information. I didn't have the courage to call the doctor (who inseminated mother) because I thought somehow I wasn't entitled to know. So I thought at least I would call the clinic to see if I could find out more about it. And it was very humiliating to call them, because they were very irate that my mother had even told me the truth. Eventually I did meet my mother's gynecologist. I finally got the nerve up to talk to this guy. I was wondering, well, is this guy my donor? There were some similarities. There were more similarities from him and me than between my dad and me. It was like I just wanted to hear his voice. I didn't want to confront him about being DI. I felt great. It felt like, this is just an ordinary guy and I could just talk to him. It wasn't scary. Part of me wants him to be my donor. You just want information that legitimately should be yours.

I was searching, trying to figure out which one of the graduate students in 1945 (was the donor). If I try to get a photograph or something in the newspaper, that's one thing, but trying to see what a person looks like, how do you make contact with somebody without making them suspicious of what you're doing? I felt like a stalker.

I worked in the same building where the Family Life History Center is and I used to go down there and see all these people searching out their roots, going back to ancestors several generations, hundreds of years prior. It's a legitimate search for them and people are given the right to know who their great-great-great-grandfather is, even though it has no significance in their daily life today. They feel that need for connection, and that's when it's felt very strong to me, that I deserve, I should have a right to know who my very first father was. I don't even have the right to know my first link on the tree.

I wondered who was this guy, that gave me life. What was his motive? Anyway, just about five or six months after I found out, I decided when I was back in town to look him (mother's doctor) up. He was dying. That was my dilemma, I didn't want to cause anybody any problems or anything. But I just wanted to know the truth. He was somewhat sympathetic. He gave me the guys (donors) name. His name was Dutch. Two weeks later, the go-between got a call from him saying, "Just tell him that he came from good genetic stock." So I was real devastated by that. It was frustrating, a lot of frustration, constant frustration.

For years our mother wanted to prattle on endlessly about her ancestors, and she had an annoying self centered way about her. But the other thought was, after I knew about this, well, I don't know who my father is yet, why don't I find him first, and then we'll deal with your ancestors. I mean, it's not that I'm not interested in her ancestors. But she couldn't grasp that she is doing research on her family tree several hundred years, while I don't know who my father is. She just couldn't quite get the unfairness and the foolishness of that.

Finding my father is still a goal. Now of course he's very possibly dead. He looked like me. My mother saw him getting off the elevator. He was tall like me, he had brown curly hair like me, and he was pulling on a hat. I wear hats a lot. This guy was my father, we think.

I wrote to many doctors and searched around. I went to the medical school and got out the books, and tried to find doctors who looked like me, and wrote tons of letters, most of which were ignored, but a few would get a patronizing response from doctors old enough to be my father. They would write back and say, well I can't help you with who your father is, but I can help you by saying you really ought to get counseling. In other words, the problem was always that if I would just not try to find my father, I would be better off. They don't get it.

My mother knew the doctor's name (who inseminated her). She knew he had died. But I couldn't find any information about him. I had gone to the library, and they actually had an obit file on little notecards of people that had died. Every time I looked him up, he wasn't in this card file, and it just really frustrated me. I still have never seen a picture of him. We went to the Probate Court, and we pulled the file. All the ones relating to the practice were stolen. They were all missing. So somebody else had been there. That was really eerie. I wanted to get to the yearbooks, because the doctor told her it was a medical student. We went to the medical school, and said that we had to look at yearbooks for some reason. I'm looking at yearbook pictures, and I couldn't tell. I just thought it was going to be so obvious that some of my features would be right there, and it was hard. I came away with a few names, but never followed through on them. It just got too emotional, too hard. My husband got a yearbook picture of one of his kids. I don't think you could rule it out certainly, the nose is a little weird. I have a picture of his daughter right here. I keep it right near my bed, it's with me. I would still love to try to find the doctor's picture.

I made my search for my donor father. When I first found out that I was a donor offspring, one of the pieces of information that my mother gave to me was that she said, "I think that the doctor who ran the clinic, it was a private clinic, and who we saw was in fact the donor." So, in a way, I already had a sort of picture of who my father might be. I had that in my mind from then on in. I was uncertain. On the one hand, I believed it. On the other hand, I was concerned because I thought probably I need to believe it. Maybe I just need to think that that's who my father was. Maybe it's better than not knowing anything. Maybe I need to believe in a fantasy. Throughout my life from then on I sort of fantasized about the possibilities of him being my father and used to go look in the phone directory to see if his clinic was still there. I just used to check him out and see if he was still there. I decided to try and make some contact. He must have been about 50 when I was conceived, so I thought the chances of him being alive were probably unlikely. I think that may have been a factor in my search. I think, at some level, I waited until he died, so that I couldn't be rejected by him...They forwarded my letter onto her (the doctor's widow.) I went to visit her. I talked to her about everything, except ask her the question as to whether she thought he might be the donor. I think I was so frightened of her saying no. I then made a decision I would face up to it. I met her daughter. She kept me at arm's length, and said that she didn't think that I looked anything like members of their family. When she said that to me, I broke down in tears. It was too much to hear that at that moment, because that was the first time somebody was rejecting me in my process. That was a very hard moment. They said, "what do you want to do?' And I said, "I feel that I would like to know for definite. I would like to be DNA tested just to rule out the possibility, or to finally decide one way or another." Within a week I had a letter from her saying we're prepared to go ahead with it. I was absolutely amazed. I was so shocked. I hadn't expected that at all. Then I got the results back and it was positive, which was just unbelievable, and very, very, very, very emotional for me. And since then I've just been making connections. It's extraordinary. Finding out seemed to be so important. Knowing seemed to be so important. I think not knowing was going to be the worst thing for me. The relief was enormous. I was absolutely ecstatic. I'm not really sure how else it's affected me. I just think a general sort of calm, a feeling of calm in relation to me, to who I am, a sense of calm.

I consciously decided that I wanted to do some more investigating about my donor father, to see if I could find who this anonymous person was, for a number of reasons. The most forefront was the realization that my daughter was becoming of age and she was going to leave home without anything about her medical background and what kind of genetically tagged diseases we might be passing on. There were some periods of time when I was doing my investigating that I would get very excited and get all these e-mails, and be writing about it and think about it. And then other times, I would just go on with my life and be fine. It wasn't any big deal.

To realize that I was not biologically part of my father's family was significant. It was disrupting. Therefore if I was able to find out what family I did belong to as far as my blood was concerned, that would be important. I would be curious to know where I fit in, in a sense.

So that was my initial attitude...governed by mostly the perception that we would just never know (the donor). There was no chance of knowing. So that is the thing that began to shift. I always thought it would be interesting and cool to know who the father was. I suppose when it became conceivable that we might track, through a combination of research and DNA testing, to track down some of the roots, it was pretty interesting, and pretty exciting. I never felt that it was this huge gap. But never the less, there's a certain lack that we feel. There's a certain sense of not having something that other people have, not knowing something. So I feel that it's not a huge agony in my life. But it would be very exciting to find out. Now I found it a pleasurable, an exciting journey, if you like, to explore the origins. That's really occupied me a lot.

What a surprising, intense experience it has been to do this quest (search for donor), and I think it jarred me at a much deeper level than I thought it would. It says something about how fundamental it is.

6. <u>Search for half-siblings, feeling a connection with them</u>

There was a desire among these donor offspring to know their half-siblings, i.e., those people who were conceived with sperm from the same donor. Donor offspring felt that there is a connection in some way to these half-siblings. There was confusion expressed about how to identify half-siblings and how to approach them. It was a common experience to be told by others that they look like someone else, or "have a twin." They felt like there were others of themselves in the world. Due to not being able to have access to accurate information about who these people are, a lot of fantasizing or assumptions occurred to try to put the unknown pieces of the genetic puzzle together.

I wonder how many of my brothers (half-siblings) have gone through the same kind of confusion and identity crises that I have, and still don't know that they are that way (DI). I just really feel sorry for them.

People come up to me and confuse me for somebody else. Every once in a while, I'll see somebody that I'll think, god, I wonder if he's my brother and not knowing whether or not I can actually have the guts to go and ask him about his origins. I just wonder constantly.

It was like watching myself almost. They said, "He very well could be your brother." And I don't know what to say. I don't know how to approach the guy, because if he doesn't know, then it would be devastating for him to find out that way. So I'm sensitive to his reaction. And if he does know, then it would be tragic, because we're too afraid to speak to each other about it. I haven't thought of a good way to solve that dilemma.

So then I started wondering about brothers and sisters. There were 18,000 records, and I found five siblings. And they were all girls. I was looking for a brother. Over the next several years, I tracked them all down the best I could. One wouldn't believe me. But the other one was our next door neighbor. There is a lot of bitterness and a lot of disappointment, even though there was no dead end. It turned out the less than happy ending for me.

Because the doctor used donors more than once, I have unknown other siblings.

All my life people were always saying to me, "Oh, you look so familiar. I just saw your twin." My mother remembers that there was an article, Life Magazine, late 60's, there's a person that looks just like me. Some neighbors noticed it, and had actually given my mother the magazine, and said, "Look, there's your daughter." So there were others of me out there. There's probably people walking around here that are related to me, other teenagers that are related to my kids. That's eerie.

I was in Chicago, and these two women came up to me and one said "Wow, we just noticed how much you look like me." I just was in such shock. I almost felt like following them out after they left, and asking them if they knew. So I was wondering if they knew and they were wondering if I knew something. Or maybe I was making too much of it. It just struck me that, after she left, maybe I should have asked her "Are you my sister?"

I saw a picture of her daughter (daughter of the gynecologist) when she was younger, and my heart nearly stopped, because she looked very like me. I desperately wanted to meet with my brother (donor's son.) I had to be very patient. It seemed a long time to me. It seemed like a lifetime. I was connected to him in some strange way.

Hunches are that there are perhaps even literally hundreds of our half siblings from the same donor father. Chances are that there are all kinds of us running around. Many people, of course, don't know, because they were never told.

We decided to have blood taken just to have DNA testing. We discovered that he indeed is our half-sibling, and therefore we all three share the some donor father. I was just totally amazed, and really excited about it, too, because I thought this is really fun to have another sibling all of a sudden, even though he's not been raised with us. But he still feels like he is part of our family, in some way. We haven't quite figured out all the rules about how you relate to somebody you meet when you're middle aged and genetically your half sibling, but you've never seen before. There aren't any rules about what you're supposed to do. So we decided we'll obviously go on and just go where the flow takes us in terms of the relationship. It's really been positive. It was probably a really emotional time for me.

It sort of blows your mind to think of all these hundreds of half siblings that could have married without knowing it, and could have been bearing children, and who knows what has happened along the way. It's kind of a strange thought to think about. And that's the reality, too.

7. <u>Concern about next generation and inherited medical conditions</u>

For some donor offspring, there was concern about not knowing what inheritable medical conditions they could have and may be passing down genetically. This issue came more into focus at turning points, such as children moving away from home, or having children or grandchildren. There were mixed viewpoints about whether it was worthwhile getting genetically tested to determine if they have genes for particular diseases.

> I had a medical condition, I had cataracts removed when I was 48, and then it hit me that this came from the donor, because it was an inherited condition and none of my maternal family have had cataracts. What else is hidden in there?

> It's really hard not knowing my history. Medically it would be lovely to know if I'm very healthy. I would love to be genetically tested.

> When it (DI) bothers me the most, is when I get asked medical questions. More after having children, it makes me wonder, because of them, because you wonder: Do they look like him? Are you passing down genes for illnesses, or things like that?

> My daughter was becoming of age and she was going to leave home and here I was letting her go without having done any kind of homework in terms of finding our for her anything about her medical background and what kind of genetically tagged diseases we might be passing on.

> The other thing that I'm real aware of, half of my genetic background is unknown. I don't think it's worth going to the university and getting all these big genetic tests, and so forth, because what would I do differently anyway. I would still just go on doing as preventative work as I could.

> At first, my position was it doesn't really matter, because medically what you do is you just get tested for everything. You just basically live healthily. You'll eventually die anyway.

8. Feeling alone as a donor offspring, having a need for contact with others and support

Initially donor offspring had difficulty finding other people with similar experiences. They felt alone in confronting their status. Finding other donor offspring and talking about their experiences was a relief.

> It was so frustrating trying to find out any information. I started to feel all alone in all of this. I didn't know anybody else like that (donor offspring), and it was very difficult to deal with, because I thought this is crazy. Am I the only one person like this? Is it right? There felt like a helplessness. There was nothing I could do...I just wanted to make contact with different people, so I wrote letters. I had finally made contact with a group. That was very helpful.

> There must be thousands of us around. For me, the most significant thing about this whole process is meeting other DI adoptees, because that more than anything validates my own feelings, because every time I talk with a new person who has contacted me, it's the same. Their experiences are almost identical in the basic feeling that mine was.

> When I finally learned about the artificial insemination group, and was able to talk to other people, I felt I was home. Talking is good, being on the same wavelength with another person. It's nice to not be completely alone.

> It was just a relief to talk to someone. I just was grateful for the woman from Donor Offspring for connecting me with people, and right after that she did a couple of conference calls. I can't tell you how helpful that was for me, because I was just having a lot of problems. So thank God for being able to talk with them. I had to talk about it. It was very important to me. My husband was helpful for me to talk it out, but certainly talking to the group was just the best. It was just so helpful for me to know that there were other people out there. It was just wonderful. I actually started keeping a little journal at the time because I realized that really was going to help me. It was like talking to people. If I couldn't talk to people, I would write it down.

> It never occurred to me that there were lots of others (donor offspring). I mean, I knew there were somewhere in my mind. It was quite a shock when she told me that she met two others. I was excited.

9. Finding support and similar experiences in adoption groups

Adoption groups provided support for some donor offspring. They found similarities in experience with adoptees.

> A significant thing for me at the same time was finding an adoption support group. Then I finally was able to talk one-on-one with, or in a group, with other people who had lived a very similar experience. I really have a very strong sense that it isn't all that much different from adoption from the point of view of the person who is the adoptee. To me the essential significance about being a DI adoptee, as is a regular adoptee, is being severed from your biological connection. I started reading a lot of adoption literature and meeting a lot of adoptees and they really understood me and validated my concerns and they validated my feelings about DI.

> There was a phone number in the paper for an adoption group. I called, and the woman was really, really supportive, and I actually went to a couple of the adoption group meetings here. They were great, and very supportive, some of the same issues. I saw a lot of people struggling, many of the same struggles, except they have a different feeling, the whole feeling of abandonment. I didn't feel abandoned.

10. Need to seek out information about donor insemination

Donor offspring felt a need to find out more information about the history and practice of donor insemination. There was also a feeling of having their own feelings validated in the literature. They also read about infertility, adoption, and eugenics.

> I looked up things in the library. Nothing was really written about DI from the point of view of the child until '87, so for four years I had no resources or anything to validate my concerns. I started doing more research into literature about infertility.

> After I found out, I always wondered what is this donor insemination stuff about. My first instinct was to look it up in the dictionary. It said used specifically in animal mating, and I thought, "Oh great! What is all this?"

> I read everything I could find about donor insemination. The best thing I did for my own psyche after finding out on a Sunday

afternoon, was I went to the library trying to find anything I can. I found my family in <u>Lethal Secrets</u>. I just had to know everything I could find and read about it. That took me a year. I think I read everything I could in the English language. I found every article he (mother's gynecologist) had ever written, so I had those kinds of basic information. In one of his articles, he talks about some of the infertile clients that he had, and I'm sure one of those is my father. There was a book translated from the Dutch, that was written around '57 or maybe early '60's, and oh my God, my mother's doctor was interviewed! He told what he did. I kept the book out a long time, but it was like one of those defining moments. I did a lot of reading about adoption. And I'd read a book. I was trying to find out information about anything they were doing with eugenics.

11. <u>Positive feelings: being special, interesting, wanted, grateful to be alive</u>

Some of the co-researchers felt special, interesting, and wanted because of being donor offspring. The feelings of being special sometimes started internally and sometimes resulted from other people treating them as special people. There was a recognition of the courage it took for their parents to do donor insemination.

Being a DI adoptee is kind of fascinating to me, because it's a new thing. It's not really a new thing, because it's so old, but it's a new thing in the public consciousness, so it's nice to be part of that consciousness raising element.

I'm as much into finding it interesting.

I'm glad I'm here, so I'm glad my parents wanted to have a child bad enough that they did that (DI).

In some senses, it makes me feel special. In some ways, I don't mind. In some ways, it's like pulling something exciting out of the cupboard, that people weren't expecting, and in some way making you quite interesting and different. So, in some ways, I have quite a positive feeling about that. It's mostly an okay kind of feeling for me.

She (the doctor's widow) said, "Oh, you're one of his babies!" She made me feel really kind of special. I think that was one of the most moving moments in my entire life, was when she made me feel a part of something, connected to something, and that I'm wanted. She said, "We were always interested in all his babies. He really loved what he was doing, and we felt it was really important. You must be very special." That made me feel unbelievably wanted. That was a lovely feeling.

In terms of feeling, I don't feel a great sorrow. I don't feel any crime has been done to me. I don't feel that I'm suffering because of it. It wasn't painful for me. I see it as being interesting, and it motivates me to action. Our mother was really good in the way that she told us, really respectful and really thoughtful. I remain grateful and admiring of both my parents for having done it. I'm glad they did. I'm glad to be alive. I admire them for having the courage at a time when it was extremely difficult, where it was basically illegal, quasi-illegal...to have the moral courage, the intellectual courage to think it through, and just the courage to do it. We know that somebody had to want us pretty much to go through that. Thank you to them.

12   Negative thoughts and feelings: troubled, angry, injustice, loss, nonexistence, split feelings

For some of the co-researchers, being a donor offspring created existential anxiety in the form of rebelling against God and a feeling of nonexistence, even before they knew they were donor offspring. There were feelings of being robbed, anger, and having many feelings at the same time.

It really screwed my head up. Trying to put my life together... certainly, it answered some questions, but it certainly created a lot more questions. I'm 28 years old, and this is all pretty new to me. I would find a little bit out at a time, and I would have to put it down. It would just eat me up inside. What kind of a world is this? I was already a rebel without a cause. Now I was a rebel with a cause. It made me so angry! It made me think the world was a pathetic place. People were pathetic. I rebelled against God. On the one hand, I just praised Him, on the other hand, I just wanted to spit in His face. I remember thinking that Lord, I don't want to be in heaven. I'd rather be in the other place. It was part of the adjusting. It took a long, long, long, long time. It's just been so difficult.

I've become cynical.

It's always been vital to me, from the moment that I was told. We were robbed. We were stolen from.

I had always been very scared of dying, because I couldn't really come to terms with my nonexistence in the world. I think part of that was to do with the fact that in some sense I didn't feel like I existed in the world, because I didn't know what half of me originated from. It was almost like that part of me had been seriously denied because of the secrecy. Nobody had spoken about it for me. So it's almost like I had come into the world by magic. So I did have a sense of not really fully being here, or being acknowledged, by my own family. In making that connection (with sperm donor's family), it made me feel complete in the fact that I really believed as though I existed. Part of what's happened is I haven't had the same panics that I used to have about death and dying. That's been quite impactful.

The wounded, and here I am reversing what I was saying earlier, saying we weren't necessarily wounded, but there is a split. I have been hurt by it. I feel many things about it, or I think many things about it. I feel I have a lack and a loss, but I don't necessarily see that as being sorrow. I see it as being a condition of my life.

13. Wanting to normalize being a donor offspring, accepting the reality

Co-researchers recognized that they went through stages in confronting the reality of being a donor offspring. After time, there was a level of integrating it as part of who they were. They normalized it as one of the many challenges people have in their lives. Current relationships took priority and helped donor offspring put this part of their lives in perspective. Some didn't think about it anymore. Some continued to work on the issues. Despite normalizing it themselves, they sometimes had to explain it to other people who were unfamiliar with it.

I still live a normal life. I'm very much into my work and into my family. We have very strong relationships, and DI doesn't obsess me. It is something I am deeply concerned about and do a lot of work on, but it doesn't keep me from living in the here and now. The thing is I do have a life.

It just doesn't matter any more. I really am thankful that I outgrew it. It took so many years, and one thing that helped is I met my wife, falling in love, and getting married, and certainly having your own children. It kind of wears off. My mother is dead. My father is dead. I don't think much about my past. I basically wasted like forty years. I'm sorry. I'm a Christian. I love the Lord. I don't question those things anymore. We all have our crosses to bear. We all have our challenges in life. My challenges certainly have been here. Most people are a lot more challenged that I am right now. God's been really, really good to me. There's a happy ending. If I tell my story, it used to take hours. It all kind of blends together now. You go through stages. I'm at 100%. It's just not even an issue in my life. That's strange. I never thought I would be in a position to say that. That's great. Things are good.

One thing you learn as you get older is that no matter how annoying or problematic something you went through is, someone else has experienced something much more horrible. Artificial insemination is dishonest, it's unfair, and it's stealing. But on the other hand, we weren't blown up by the Oklahoma bomber. It really is something you need to keep in perspective.

Our circumstance was different. A lot of people have different circumstances. (e.g. born out of wedlock, one night stand.) It does goof people up. At least we were born out of love, and they were, too, but I think it's different. At least they can know who the father is. Most people don't have your typical family life, the father knows best kind of family life. It's always some sort of secret in every family. Maybe it's just my group of friends.

When I've talked about it in conversation to friends, the thing I've always noticed is the feeling that I'm imparting some mementous piece of information to somebody else, but at the same time wanting to be very normal about it and for it to be very normal and nothing exceptional. Yet I feel that it always is something exceptional. I'm waiting for the "oh, wow, what is that?" or "gosh, what a surprise!" I've always wanted to impart it in as casual and natural way as possible. I was trying to normalize the fact that I was a donor offspring and for it not to be something that was so part of my life that I was talking about it continuously. Perhaps inside of me I had normalized it. I didn't feel it was so normal for other people when they heard it. There was a dichotomy between how I might perceive it and how others might perceive it. It always led to a much more in depth conversation about being a donor offspring, because other people were so unfamiliar with it. It's this sense of I'm going to have to deal with this, they're going to talk about it, and I need to make it as open as possible for them, so that they feel comfortable with it, so it doesn't in any way get in the way of what's going on between us.

14. Developed beliefs that knowledge of genetic and medical history are a birthright

As a result of confronting being a donor offspring, both from their inner struggles and from their research into donor insemination, donor offspring developed strong beliefs about their rights as donor offspring. They felt that their rights included knowledge of the truth about who their biological parents were and knowledge of their medical history. There was a belief among some of the co-researchers that donor insemination was a form of eugenics.

> They (clinic staff) said I had no right to know my medical history. That really hit me hard. I actually called the ACLU and they said there is no legal recourse. There is no precedence about trying to find this. It was so frustrating.

> When I asked my mom why couldn't dad have kids, she told me that he was sterilized. He was at the state home, they were called Homes for Feeble Minded Youth, and they did it. Then I do research and I found out about eugenics and artificial insemination. DI is a form of eugenics, because they certainly don't use dumb people. They use the best and the brightest. I think they did it innocently. It's just sort of innocent stupidity, wishful thinking.

> I didn't want to cause anybody any problems or anything. I just wanted to know the truth. I think I had a right as a human being to know who my biological provider was.

> I just don't think it's fair that we would never be able to really know who he (donor) is, that it's so secretive. Our parents or the doctors and everybody involved just didn't really consider what the children

would think about it. They just thought about a little baby, not what they were going to be like as adults, or wonder when they're adults.

I think that I came to see it as more of a right than a need. The basic situation that applies to 95% of people on the planet is that they know who their genetic forebears were as a matter of course, as part of the hand of cards they get, as part of their birthright. If you're going to deprive us of that information when it's in your power to give it to us, and if you're going to advocate secrecy and lying and deception, then you better justify what you're doing. There is no real justification for it. I always feel that we're kind of pushed into a position of being victims and being wounded in order to be given the information and the knowledge.

The article said nine people out of 45,000 have tried to go through the courts to find out their identity, as though that were evidence. If it was a matter of life and death, perhaps we would all launch court cases. You know what civil action is, what a nightmare it would be, how much money it would take, and how much pain it would be. It's so ridiculous. It's extremely annoying to read stuff like that., because these are the same people whose practice is founded on genetics. It's a bit hypocritical for them to say that it is unimportant when the science upon which they based their craft is screaming it's importance all the time, increasingly every day. It is also ridiculous because our entire culture is geared towards it. Finding roots and genealogy is an obsessive industry. It's right throughout the culture. There's a thousand stories about people trying to find their true father. It's a continual human narrative.

15. Becoming an activist, finding a sense of purpose, duty to speak up

The co-researchers felt a need to speak out about being a donor offspring. They did this in different ways—in the media, to groups of DI parents, or more anonymously. To some, speaking out about DI became a mission to help improve the rights of other donor offspring. A need for regulation of donor insemination was expressed. As the field of genetics expands, the experiences of donor offspring were viewed as becoming more important to pay attention to.

I had a dream, and this was kind of a key dream in my whole process of dealing with DI, where I was going. I decided that, analyzing that dream, that what it was telling me is that I had a duty to speak out, if not for my own good, I had an obligation to all the other people being conceived through DI. It was really the pivot point where I changed into an activist. People were calling me up from everywhere. I started feeling stronger and stronger about my crusade to educate DI parents that they needed to understand who we are, and what their children will go through. I feel really a strong sense of purpose there, and that really is very encouraging, or really validating for me that actually now I have people finally listen to me. I'm just speaking out about a social concern that I think very few people are aware of..

I had decided to go public with my story. I went on this talk radio show, Merv Griffin, Hard Copy, Jeraldo. That was disappointing. Joan Rivers was interesting. I had no regrets of what happened. Then I started getting more in the political thing, wanting to help people, and get rid of these anonymous sperm banks that create anonymous people. I'm sure that I had some impact on it, but I don't think about it any more. That's great for me, maybe not for the cause of DI offspring or adoptees.

I think what's important is that artificial insemination as normally practiced is a lie. We could be doing things, but we would need to have unity. It's nothing I can do alone. I joined an adoption group for quite a few years before I learned about the artificial insemination group, but the motto is "the right to the truth of our origins." In other words, let's stop lying. Let's have rules that say that when the child turns eighteen, there will be a meeting with the probate judge, the file will be open, everything will be shown, and pictures will be shown, there will be visits allowed with all of the parents, whoever they are, where ever they are, and if you don't like that, then don't participate. My message is you do whatever you want (in infertility treatments), we'll license all these different things, but it's going to be done professionally, and the truth is going to be told. It's going to be regulated. We'll have it, but we will regulate it.

At different times, the Donor Offspring leader would send journalists my way. I felt that it should be talked about and it should be in the open, but since my mother was still alive, I just didn't feel like suddenly appearing on 20/20 or something like that, so I never did any of that. I did do an English newspaper article a year or two later.

I've done any survey that's come my way. I try to do everything I can, sort of anonymously at this point.

Now that people are more accepting of it, I think it's important for those people that are thinking about doing it, that they need to consider the long run of the child, and to be honest with them about it. I think it's good that they get more information now about the donor, about their medical history, and what they are like. We don't have that at all.

I went and spoke. The people were either recipients of donor sperm, or they were thinking about using DI as a fertility treatment, or mothers who were pregnant. Unbelievable! Very, very empowering. I was amazed that I could speak for 45 minutes even without written notes. I just spoke. That was a good feeling. I was absolutely overwhelmed by the response I got. A lot of people stood up at the end. People were in tears. They were obviously very, very moved by the story, which I thought was just amazing. It was a big thing to speak out like that, to be accepted for what it was I was speaking out about.

A journalist talked to me on the phone, during the time I started to do my research, and interviewed me and got my thoughts and ideas, that she then contributed to her comments that were made on the program.

I'm a supporter of disclosure with kids right from the beginning. I don't see why there shouldn't be laws put into effect, like there are for adoption, where there's a registry that tells about donor fathers, so that then children of donors can find out about their donor father in the future, when they get to be of age.

I really would like to help future families. I've been a therapist. Now I've become more aware of the whole issues that have affected me as a person. I wouldn't mind going around and at least consulting with other therapists or other professionals who are working with couples who are going to use DI, just to encourage them to make sure that the families have as healthy an attitude about this whole thing as they can in terms of raising the kids in as healthy an environment, and to not just think of the pregnancy aspect. I think so many infertile couples are so focused on the very beginning stages of birth and having a baby, that they sort of forget that this is a person that is going to grow up and have a whole life. Their job is to guide and help that person to be who they are and to celebrate who they are as a person and as an individual. Anyone who is working in those kind of clinics, I think needs to be aware of all those things. So if I can do anything to help people along that way, I will.

It's a discontinuity, it's a dissonance, and it gives me the desire to speak the way I have been speaking, which I do, and it gives me the desire to have a public voice about this and try to make these kind of points. It is personal, too. I don't want to suggest that my animus, that the energy that's driving this is not personal. Of course it is. It is a very personal thing, but I also think that we have an opportunity, reproductive technology children, to raise these kind of issues, to be a mirror. We are evidence, and so are adoptees, although we are in a different way, because we have one genitor and one not genitor. Because our make up is split, then we provide a kind of a window or a mirror on these functions. It's not just that. It's also that we're on the threshold of a time when we have the power to manipulate genetics. I think that the offspring of every productive technology are important people to listen to because of what's coming. Our experience is going to be significant, because it is the experience of possibly many more people to come. If we start to break the genetic links between children and their genitors, if we start to manipulate those links, if we start to design people, the needs and experiences of offspring are going to become more and more in evidence.

Textural Description

From the themes, I developed a composite textural description. This is the final stage of the phenomenological reduction. I took the data and themes and focused it into a description of what the meaning of the experience of confronting the reality of being a donor offspring is for the co-researchers in this study.

These donor offspring uniformly felt that it is best to know, from an early age, of being a donor offspring. Secrecy created alliances in their families. The revelation of being a donor offspring made sense to them. Some offspring had an earlier intuition that their fathers were not their biological fathers. There was difficulty in telling other people about being donor offspring, because others did not understand its importance and relevance, unless they were offspring or adoptees themselves.

Identity issues were fundamental for donor offspring. Even before knowing that they were donor offspring, there was confusion about why they were different from other family members in some ways. Knowing and understanding themselves as donor offspring was an important part of clarifying their identities.

Donor offspring experienced a desire for ancestral connection and to know who their sperm donor was. Without this information, they fantasized about characteristics of the donor. There was also a desire to know their half-siblings, those people who were conceived with sperm from the same donor. It was a common experience to be told that they look like other people, and then wonder if they were half-siblings.

Some donor offspring were concerned about what inheritable medical conditions are in their unknown genes. This especially came into focus during family turning points, such as children being born or leaving home.

Donor offspring initially felt alone in confronting the reality of being donor offspring. Finding other offspring and talking about their experiences was a great relief. Adoption support groups also provided support for some donor offspring. They found similar experiences and understanding from adoptees.

Donor offspring also sought information about the history and process of donor insemination. There was a validation of their own feelings in literature from the point of view of the offspring. Donor offspring also read about infertility, adoption, and eugenics, as related topics to donor insemination.

Confronting the reality of being a donor offspring brought out a whole array of strong feelings for donor offspring. Some of the positive emotions experienced were a feeling of being special and interesting, being wanted, and being grateful to be alive. There was a recognition of the courage it took for their parents to use donor insemination. Some of the negative feelings were being troubled, angry, strong feelings of injustice and loss, and existential loss due to not knowing part of one's identity.

In confronting the reality of being donor offspring, people went through stages. There was an integration of being a donor offspring as part of who they were, part of their identity. Some offspring normalized the experience as one of many challenges people face in life. Initially, there was an obsession about the ramifications of being a donor offspring.

Priorities refocused back to current relationships as donor offspring put this part of their life into perspective.

Donor offspring developed strong beliefs about their rights to knowledge of the truth about their biological parents and to such things as their genetic medical history. Some donor offspring felt a duty to speak out about donor insemination to help improve the rights of all donor offspring. A need for regulation of donor insemination was seen.

IMAGINATIVE VARIATION

The goal of imaginative variation was to find the essence of the experience. I looked at the experience of confronting the reality of being a donor offspring with reference to the seven universal structures: spatiality, temporality, materiality, causality, bodily awareness, relationship to self, and relationship to others. I supported each of these areas with quotes from the co-researchers.

From this study of the structures, I then developed a composite structural description of the experience of confronting the reality of being a donor offspring.

Universal Structures

1. Spatiality

Donor offspring's comments relating to spatial relationships focused on closeness and distance in relationships, and wondering where they came from and how they fit into the world. The secrecy of donor insemination for them created a distance between father and child. They believed that DI should be in the open. There was a feeling of being severed from biological connections and not fully being here. Being a donor offspring is central to oneself.

A secret is definitely a barrier to closeness in the family.

I would say, "Where did I come from?"

Everything revolves around my mother.

My father had a relatively removed kind of a fathering style. I think he felt remote from me.

I think it (DI) turned the relationship (between parents) around.

It seemed like a greater part of me just came out of the blue.

I'm a donor offspring. I had no idea it was so central to who I was.

I have a picture of his (mother's doctor) daughter right here. I keep it right near my bed. It's with me.

Since then I've just been making connections.

I would be curious to know where I fit in (genetically).

I never felt that it was this huge gap.

To me the essential significance about being a DI adoptee is being severed from your biological connection.

I'm glad I'm here (born).

That was one of the most moving moments in my entire life, was when she made me feel a part of something, connected to something, and that I'm wanted.

We know that somebody had to want us pretty much to go through that.

I remember thinking that Lord, I don't want to be in heaven. I'd rather be in the other place.

It's almost like I had come into the world by magic. So I did have a sense of not really fully being here.

It was really the pivot point where I changed into an activist.

I felt that it (DI) should be talked about and it should be in the open.

2. Temporality

Confronting the reality of being a donor offspring was a process of adjustment. It took time. Sometimes people waited to confront a part of the experience until they felt ready to handle it. At times, one second was vital, a revelation, e.g., the moment of finding out about being a donor offspring. Time sometimes separated connections with people or brought them together.

The second our mother told me, it made massive sense.

We talked about it for the first time ever.

"I'm a donor offspring," was the very first thing that came out. I couldn't be me without telling her that first.

It was really kind of an amazing time (finding out about DI).

They had told me they destroyed the records after seven years.

People are given the right to know who their great-great-great-grandfather is, even though it has no significance in their daily life today. I should have a right to know who my very first father was.

I assumed he (donor) would be in his late nineties, so I thought the chances of him being alive were probably unlikely. I think, at some level, I waited until he died, so that I couldn't be rejected by him.

It was too much to hear that at that moment, because that was the first time somebody was rejecting me in my process. That was a very hard moment.

I thought if I'm going to do any of this kind of investigating, I better hurry up and do it now. My donor father might be no longer living.

My initial attitude was governed by the perception that there was no chance of knowing. That is the thing that began to shift.

It seemed a long time to me (meeting donor's son). It seemed a lifetime. Since then, it's just been a slow process of acknowledgment. I think the changes in me are very slow and very gradual and probably will carry on making changes to my life.

This is really fun to have another sibling all of a sudden.

I think there will be some times in the future, particularly when my children start to have their own children, that these issues will start to hit me even stronger again.

At first, my position (re: medical history) was it doesn't really matter. You'll eventually die anyway.

It (DI) is at least thousands of years old. It is quite a bit older than people realize, but it's a new thing in the public consciousness.

After finding out on a Sunday afternoon.

It (DI) doesn't keep me from living in the here and now.

I don't think much about my past. I basically wasted like forty years. There's a happy ending. If I tell my story, it used to take hours. It all kind of blends together now.

They (parents and doctors) just thought about a little baby, not what they were going to be like as adults, or wonder when they're adults.

Let's have rules that when the child turns eighteen, the file will be open.

I don't see why there shouldn't be laws put into effect, like there are for adoption, where there's a registry that tells about donor fathers, so that then children of donors can find out about their donor father in the future, when they get to be of age.

3. Materiality

Donor offspring spoke of having their genetic history stolen from them. There was a loss of something, their roots, that other people have. There was a realization of having to confront the hand of cards they were dealt. Donor offspring saw themselves as a window or mirror for others to understand what the experience of being a child of a reproductive technology is like.

It was a reaction of having the rug pulled out from under you.

It (artificial insemination) is stealing. It is injustice, unfairness, we've been robbed.

SPERM DONOR OFFSPRING:

If you step off and you're not perfect children, slap you across the face and make you feel guilty.

I kept the code of silence.

A father sees this other man (donor) reflected in the boy.

It (DI) just drove a wedge between them (parents) really.

It's just not knowing what your roots are.

So what if I came from a turkey baster, or whatever.

I used to go down there and see all these people searching out their roots. I don't even have the right to know my first link on the tree.

Medical school, yearbooks, pictures, books, letters, library, newspapers, DNA test, research, records, website, internet, registry, conference calls, journal, medical history, information, studies, license, regulate.

Maybe it's better than not knowing anything. Maybe I need to believe in a fantasy.

It's in your interest to get on with your life with the cards you have dealt. So it is with DI. But never the less, there's a certain lack that we feel. There's a certain sense of not having something that other people have, not knowing something.

The DI business was really something I did have to confront.

These books validated my feelings, because they really did look into what it is like for a person born through DI and what they go through.

When I finally learned about the artificial insemination group, and was able to talk to other people, I felt I was home.

Artificial insemination is not a high tech operation.

In some ways, it (telling about DI) is like pulling something exciting out of the cupboard.

I don't feel any crime has been done to me.

I couldn't really come to terms with my nonexistence in the world. In making that connection (with sperm donor's family), it made me feel complete in the fact that I really believed as though I existed.

I feel a lack and a loss. I see it as being a condition of my life.

We all have our crosses to bear.

I didn't want to cause anybody any problems. I just wanted to know the truth. I think I had a right as a human being to know who my biological provider was.

The language of rights is quite different than the language of needs. The basic situation of 95% of people on the planet is that they know who their genetic forebears were as a matter of course, as part of the hand of cards they get, as part of their birthright. Your birthright includes knowing who your genetic father was, your genitor. If you're going to deprive us of that information when it's in your power to give it to us.

Finding roots and genealogy is an obsessive industry. It's throughout the culture. There's a thousand stories about people trying to find their true father.

Then I started getting more in the political thing, wanting to help people and get rid of these anonymous sperm banks that create anonymous people.

Sperm inseminations, as one of the guys from England says. Nobody was being a donor. She's paying big bucks.

I also think that we have an opportunity, reproductive technology children, to raise these kind of issues, to be a mirror. We are evidence. We provide a kind of a window or a mirror on these functions. It's also that we're on the threshold of a time when we have the power to manipulate genetics. I think that the offspring of every productive technology are important people to listen to because of what's coming. If we start to break the genetic links between children and their genitors, if we start to manipulate those links, if we start to design people, the needs and experiences of offspring are going to become more and more in evidence.

4. Causality

There were strong feelings that being a donor offspring and confronting that reality has effects on the offspring. The secrecy affects the marital and family relationships. Finding out about being a donor offspring is the revelation which explains a lot of things in donor offspring's lives. Things then make sense. The frustration in not being able to find out information causes an obsessiveness to try to find out, e.g., who the donor is. Confronting the reality of being a donor offspring motivates people to action.

> If you're keeping it a secret, then that's going to have effects in the family. The parents know, and it's going to affect them and their interaction, and the father's going to know. And if you aren't talking about it, then why aren't you talking about it? Well, because you think it's a problem. And if you think it's a problem, then it's affecting the family. It's there in your mind, bunging up communication.

> I just thought more about how it (DI) has affected the relationship that my parents had. I think it did affect their relationship, and then affect us, too.

> The culmination of privacy, secrecy, and then withholding information—it's the combination of all those factors which affected their relationship (parents), and therefore affected the family dynamics.

> Certainly that (DI) was the revelation, in a sense, which explained everything—why I'm so very different.

> The process of therapy was part of the discovery about exactly what it had meant to me and what effects it had on me.

> It (being half Jewish genetically) totally explains a lot of things to me. It explains my emotional expressiveness.

> I immediately started searching or started trying to figure out who

the guy was. That became a bit obsessive, and so the impact of that was pretty strong, because it was so frustrating trying to find out any information.

The process of therapy was the jumping block for which I actually made my search for my donor father.

Then I got the results back (of DNA test) and it was positive, which was just unbelievable, and very, very, very, very emotional for me.

I see it (being a donor offspring) as being interesting, and it motivates me to action.

I was already a rebel without a cause. Now I was a rebel with a cause. It (confronting being a donor offspring) made me so angry!.

I've been a therapist. Now (confronting being a donor offspring) I've become more aware of the whole issues that have affected me as a person.

5. Bodily Awareness

Donor offspring said they felt different than other people and different than their parents. Physically, they were different from their father. There were hunches about who they were. There was discussion of feeling split, discontinuous, having a line drawn down the middle of themselves, or wondering what else was hidden inside of themselves. There was a focus on body parts and trying to figure out which came from the donor genetically. Confronting the reality of being a donor offspring involved accepting all of the parts of themselves and the situation. There were a lot of bodily reactions in relation to possible relationships with donors or half-siblings, and having the nerve or guts to ask people about this. There were a lot of bodily metaphors in the language of feelings of confronting the reality of being a donor offspring. It felt good to speak and be listened to about their experiences as donor offspring.

It finally was exhilarating to see what the secret was. It wasn't a shock so much, because it made sense to me. In fact, I thought it was quite liberating.

SPERM DONOR OFFSPRING:

I felt different. Unless you're an adopted person, you don't know what it feels like.

There is a difference between myself and other people.

I'm very different than my parents. And I see things differently, very differently.

I still was fairly uncomfortable with it. I think I became more bold because everyone shared so much of themselves with me. So I started being more open, too.

I touched on some kind of a nerve from the inheritance business. When I was five I had asked my mother if I was adopted and so even at that age I was aware that I wasn't like my dad.

Between my father and me, we had absolutely nothing physical in common.

I asked them (parents) what kind of blood they had. What they did was they brushed me off and they said they didn't know.

She's a spitting image of my mother. I always used to think that we had been switched.

I felt I should keep the secret for our mother. But I sort of chafed under it.

I still feel like there's a line drawn down the half of me, and I know one half, and the other half is just this other person that I can only identify that she's left handed, she talks too much, she's outgoing, all these little idiosyncrasies that are totally different than the rest of the family.

You're going around with a lot of hunches about who you are.

My brother and I, who was there, and my mom, all of us were looking at each other. He and I were particularly looking at each other, and looking at my mom, and trying to figure out—you know, looking at lengths of fingers, and looking at facial characteristics, and trying to figure out what parts of us belong to this strange new person (sperm donor) who'd kind of come into our lives. Of course, you can't isolate noses, or mouths, or ears, or whatever, because half of us come from our mother genetically.

You think about turkey basters and people masturbating in the next room, and taking the sperm and putting it into the vagina, all very clinical and sort of scientific. I think that's probably why there was part of me that was just a little uncomfortable with the whole thing, and sort of feeling weird about it.

As I got closer to 50, I personally feel an increasing sense of comfort as to who I am and embracing all the parts and then confronting the thoughts about it and realizing that that's okay.

What a surprising, intense experience it has been to do this quest, and I think it jarred me at a much deeper level that I thought it would.

I finally got the nerve up to talk to this guy. I was wondering, is this guy my donor?.

The go-between got a call from him (donor) saying, "Just tell him that he came from good genetic stock."

I'm looking at yearbook pictures (looking for donor), and I couldn't tell. I just thought it was going to be so obvious that some of my features would be right there, and it was hard.

I couldn't bring myself to ask this question as to whether she thought he might be the donor. I think I was so frightened of her saying no. I then made a decision I would face up to it. I met her daughter. She kept me at arm's length, and said that she didn't think that I looked anything like members of their family. When she said that to me, I broke down in tears.

Finding out (who donor was) seemed to be so important. Knowing seemed to be so important. The relief was enormous. I was absolutely ecstatic. I just think a general sort of calm, a feeling of calm.

To realize that I was not biologically part of my father's family was significant. It was disrupting. Therefore, if I was able to find out what family I did belong to as far as my blood was concerned, that would be important.

SPERM DONOR OFFSPRING:

I tend to believe that there are a lot of possibilities open to us. There is not a fate written in the genes. It's not deterministic. I found it a pleasurable, an exciting journey to explore the origins. That's really occupied me a lot.

I wonder how many of my brothers (half-siblings) have gone through the same kind of confusion and identity crises that I have.

Every once in a while, I'll see somebody that I'll think, god, I wonder if he's my brother and not knowing whether or not I can actually have the guts to go and ask him about his origins.

It just struck me that, after she left, maybe I should have asked her "Are you my sister?"

I saw a picture of her daughter when she was younger, and my heart nearly stopped, because she looked very like me.

It sort of blows your mind to think of all these hundreds of half siblings.

It was an inherited medical condition and none of my maternal family have had cataracts. What else is hidden in there?.

After having children, you wonder: Do they look like him? Are you passing down genes for illnesses?.

Talking is good, being on the same wavelength with another person.

The adoption group meetings were great, and very supportive.

In some senses, it makes me feel special.

It wasn't painful for me.

It really screwed up my head.

It would just eat me up inside.

In some sense I didn't feel like I existed in the world, because I didn't know what half of me originated from. It was almost like that part of me had been seriously denied because of the secrecy.

What's happened is I haven't had the same panics that I used to have about death and dying.

There is a split. I have been hurt by it.

I really am thankful that I outgrew it. It kind of wears off.

I've always wanted to impart it in as casual and natural way as possible.

I think I had a right as a human being to know who my biological provider was.

I always feel that we're kind of pushed into a position of being victims and being wounded in order to be given the information and the knowledge.

I started feeling stronger and stronger about my crusade to educate DI parents that they needed to understand who we are, and what their children will go through.

I feel really a strong sense of purpose there, and that really is very encouraging, or really validating for me that actually now I have people finally listen to me.

I just spoke. That was a good feeling. I was absolutely overwhelmed by the response I got. It was a big thing to speak out like that, to be accepted for what it was I was speaking out about.

I think so many infertile couples are so focused on the very beginning stages of birth and having a baby, that they sort of forget that this is a person that is going to grow up and have a whole life.

It's a discontinuity, it's a dissonance, and it gives me the desire to speak the way I have been speaking, which I do, and it gives me the desire to have a public voice about this.

Our make up is split.

6. Relationship to self

Being a donor offspring was part of who the co-researchers were, part of their identity. Finding out about being a donor offspring created a need to readjust their self-concept or image of who they were. Some donor offspring had self worth problems. Finding out who the donor was created a feeling of calm in relation to the self.

> We (self and siblings) all have a self respect problem or a self worth problem.

> When my mother told me (about DI), I had to go through a major readjustment of my self-concept, self-image.

> "What is this donor insemination stuff about?" I thought that I was really weird. I said, "Who am I?" I was very confused.

> I've always been pretty comfortable with who I am, and the different facets of who I am. But, of course, that means then accepting the fact that I am the offspring of an unknown donor.

> I'm still me and I'm still happy with who I am.

> It is a part of who I am.

> A feeling of calm in relation to me, to who I am (after finding our who donor is).

> So I started calling myself an adoptee.

> I was trying to normalize the fact that I was a donor offspring and for it not to be something that was so part of my life that I was talking about it continuously. Perhaps inside of me I had normalized it.

> It is personal, too. I don't want to suggest that my animus, that the energy that's driving this (speaking out) is not personal. Of course it is. It is a very personal thing.

7. Relationship to others

Donor offspring expressed feeling alone in their families and feeling alone in this experience because of initially not being able to find other donor offspring. There was a strong need to talk to other people about it—other donor offspring, other family members, friends. There was discomfort talking about being a donor offspring when people didn't understand the meaning it carries.

There was sometimes a sensing that their father was not their biological father before being told about the donor insemination. The mother was described as the dominant parent and the father as the weak parent. It was unspoken that the children were the mother's children and a feeling that the father did not like them in some way. Closeness in sibling relationships varied, related to similarities with the siblings. Relationships with spouses and their own children were close and vitally important.

Donor offspring expressed feeling a belonging in some way to the donor. They desired knowledge of the donor. For those people who had found half siblings, they felt like family to them. There was some confusion about how to relate to new found family members.

It was a common experience to look like or be mistaken for other people. The language donor offspring used indicates a feeling that there were others of themselves in the world.

Donor offspring felt a duty to speak out about their experience for the sake of future offspring. There was a need for unity among donor offspring in order to have an impact. Learning from the experience of donor offspring was seen as important, especially as more people in our society are created in situations where their social parents are not their genitors.

I felt like a stranger in my own family. I felt so totally alienated or alone in my family, even though I think that the family dynamics were fairly strong.

I wanted to tell my kids, who were teenagers at the time.

I was sitting in the kitchen one day talking to my mother, and the subject of my relationship with my father came up as it did quite often. And I just kind of knew, and I just thought I'm going to ask now whether he is actually my father, because I had sensed that he wasn't.

During our upbringing, our mother was very dominant, especially with respect to us, and our father was very much a weak member, and nothing was ever said, but it was sort of the "these are my children, I'll make decisions here" kind of a setting.

As far as parenting, then the social father is the father. He's the guy you make the connection with. My father, I never had the feeling he liked me very much. When I look back on it, after I knew about the donor insemination, it made sense, because I don't think he really felt like he was my father.

It became so obvious that what we have in our family is a major disrespect problem, which is what our mother started.

I've never felt that I had a close relationship with my sister. We're very different.

We're pretty close siblings. I feel really close to my brother, have been feeling increasingly close to my brother during this whole investigation, because he and I share that. And we're both kind of in it together.

Because I had kept it (DI) secret for quite a long time, or it just wasn't talked about, that told me that there was part of me that had some feelings about it, some discomfort perhaps, in sharing it with people. I wouldn't use as strong a word as shame, but discomfort probably.

There's a certain part of me, my identity, that feels like I do have some belonging to that other person (donor) who made me, in some way. I feel as if I would like to know who that person is. I'm just curious, what their life has been like, what their interests are, whether they have some similar characteristics as I do, which is possible, and maybe likely even—not so much how I look, but more like what internally goes on inside me and how that relates to this other person whose sperm I might come from.

Finding my father (donor) is still a goal.

People come up to me and confuse me for somebody else. Every once in a while, I'll see somebody that I'll think, god, I wonder if he's my brother. There is a person who I'm trying to find out more about who supposedly is my twin. Somebody has told me that person looks exactly like me.

Listening to the second son speak, it was like watching myself almost. We're too afraid to speak to each other about it (possibility of being half brothers).

I was connected to him (donor's son) in some strange way.

He (half brother) is part of our family, in some way. We haven't quite figured out all the rules about how you relate to somebody you meet when you're middle aged and genetically your half sibling but you've never seen before.

I started to feel all alone in all of this. I didn't know anybody else like that (donor offspring). Am I the only one person like this? I just wanted to make contact with different people. I had finally made contact with a group. That was very helpful. A significant thing for me at the same time was finding an adoption support group. For me, the most significant thing about this whole process is meeting other DI adoptees, because that more than anything validates my own feelings.

It was just a relief to talk to someone. I just was grateful for the woman from Donor Offspring for connecting me with people.

I'm very much into my work and into my family. We have very strong relationships.

One thing that helped (confront DI) is I met my wife, falling in love, and getting married, and certainly having your own children.

She (the doctor's widow) said, "Oh, you're one of his babies!".

I rebelled against God.

When I've talked about it in conversation to friends, the thing I've always noticed is the feeling that I'm imparting some momentous piece of information to somebody else. It always led to a much more in depth conversation about being a donor offspring, because other people were so unfamiliar with it. It's this sense of I'm going to have to deal with this. They're going to talk about it, and I need to make it as open as possible for them so that they feel comfortable with it, so it doesn't in any way get in the way of what's going on between us.

I had a duty to speak out, if not for my own good, I had an obligation to all the other people being conceived through DI.

Getting the medical center to cooperate and be good to us would require a group. In other words, we could be doing things, but we would need to have unity. It's nothing I can do alone.

Our experience is going to be significant, because it is the experience of possibly many more people to come.

Structural Description

From the universal structures, I developed a composite structural description. This was the final stage of the imaginative variation. I took the data and the universal structures and focused it into the essence of the experience of confronting the reality of being a donor offspring.

Donor offspring felt a distance between themselves and their fathers. They felt alone in their families. There were hunches that they did not fit in their families or that their father was not their biological father.

There was also a feeling of being severed from biological connections. They wondered how they fit in the world. Donor offspring felt that donor insemination should be done in the open. Secrecy affected the marital and family relationships. The balance of power shifted in the marital relationship. Mothers were described as dominant and fathers as weak.

Confronting the reality of being a donor offspring was an adjustment process which went through stages and took time. Finding out about being a donor offspring brought a sense of relief. At that moment, everything suddenly made sense. Their hunches about discontinuities in their life were validated.

Donor offspring felt that knowing their biological father was their birthright, and this was stolen from them. There was a loss of their roots. They felt a connection to the sperm donor and that half-siblings were family. They had to confront the reality of the cards they were dealt. The frustration in not being allowed information about the donor led to an obsessiveness to find out. Finding one's donor created a feeling of calm within themselves. Donor offspring were often told they look like other people, and felt that there were others of themselves in the world.

Donor offspring felt different from other people. They felt split, and wondered what unknown things were hidden inside of them that might have been inherited from the donor. Confronting this involved acceptance of all of the parts of themselves.

Being a donor offspring was central to who one was. It was a part of their identity. Finding out about being a donor offspring created a need to readjust their self-concept.

Confronting the realities of this situation motivated people to action. It felt good to talk about and be heard about their experiences as donor offspring. Donor offspring felt a duty to speak out to increase public awareness of the realities of being raised by non-biological parents, with secrecy about their origins. As more people will be created and raised in situations where social parents are not the genitors, the voice of donor offspring can reveal important lessons in this experience.

SYNTHESIS

The synthesis combined the meaning and essence of the textural and structural descriptions into a final description of the experience of confronting the reality of being a donor offspring.

Confronting the reality of being a donor offspring was a process and it took time. When one was told of being a donor offspring, there was usually an intense initial reaction, with emotions ranging from shock, exhilaration, liberation, to anger and embarrassment. There was a relief in knowing that hunches about not fitting in the family or their father not being their biological father were accurate. Donor offspring felt alone and different in their families. It made sense that they were donor offspring.

Secrecy affected the marital and family relationships. Donor offspring felt that it would be best to know, from an early age, about being a donor offspring.

Being a donor offspring was part of who one was, a fundamental part of their identity. Finding out and understanding themselves as donor offspring was an important part of clarifying their identities.

Donor offspring experienced a desire for ancestral connection and roots, and to know who their sperm donor and half-siblings were. They felt that this information was their birthright. They wondered how they fit in the world. Frustration in not having this information caused fantasizing about their donor and half-siblings, and an obsessiveness to find out about them. Finding one's donor created a feeling of calm within themselves.

Donor offspring were often told that they looked like other people. They wondered if these people were half-siblings. They felt like there were others of themselves in the world.

Donor offspring felt split, discontinuous, and wondered what unknown things were hidden in them that were inherited from the donor. They were concerned about unknown genetic medical conditions. This came into focus during family transitions, such as children being born or moving away from home.

Donor offspring felt alone in confronting the realities of being donor offspring. Finding other offspring and talking about their experiences was a great relief. Adoption support groups also provided support, as adoptees had similar experiences and therefore understood the experience of being raised by a non-biological parent.

Donor offspring also sought information about the history and process of donor insemination. They found validation of their feelings in literature from the point of view of the offspring.

Donor offspring developed strong beliefs about their rights to knowledge of the truth of their origins and genetic history. They were motivated to action. They felt a duty to speak out about their experience in order to help improve the rights of all people raised by non-biological parents. A need for regulation of reproductive technologies ensuring offspring rights was seen.

Confronting the reality of being a donor offspring caused a spectrum of strong feelings. Some positive emotions experienced were feeling special and interesting, being wanted, and being grateful to be alive. Some negative feelings were being troubled and angry. There were feelings of injustice and loss and existential loss due to not knowing part of one's identity.

Offspring normalized the experience as one of many challenges people face in life. Initially, there was an obsession about the ramifications of being a donor offspring. Priorities refocused back to current relationships as donor offspring put this part of their life into perspective and embraced being a donor offspring as a part of who they were. Some donor offspring felt a need to let go of this part of their lives. Others continued seeking out their sperm donor and half-siblings and were activists in fighting for the rights of all donor offspring.

CHAPTER VII
IMPLICATIONS AND APPLICATIONS

In this chapter, I describe the implications and applications of the research data. I review how this information can be applied in personal, clinical, educational, societal, policy making and legislative arenas. I also make suggestions for further research in the area of donor insemination, in particular related to the experience of donor offspring.

The knowledge and understanding of psychological implications of the practice of donor insemination is very much in evolution today. Greater sharing of personal experience by families and offspring is changing the ideology about the relevance of the situation to the parties involved, the rights and obligations, and the psychological impact. This, in turn, influences the paradigm and practice of donor insemination. As donor insemination families step forward and become less private about their experience, there is an opportunity to research what this experience has been for them and what they feel could be done to make improvements within donor conceived families and in their interactions with the world outside of the family.

Research regarding the experience of donor offspring is vital. John Lantos, M.D. concurs, stating "research on the outcomes of new reproductive technologies from the perspective of the children produced is essential" (Stotland, 1990, p. 95). In their chapter, Psychiatric Research and the New Reproductive Technologies, Jennifer Downey, M.D. and Mary McKinney, M.A., state:

> Among the affected individuals who need to be studied are the offspring of successful fertility treatment...Children conceived by donor insemination are also at risk for later psychological sequelae because of family secrecy concerning their parentage and the sense of deficit experienced by their nongenetic fathers. (Stotland, 1990, pp. 164-165)

Historically, donor offspring have not had a voice at all. The donor insemination process occurs before they are born. The contracts are written with concern for the parties involved at the time, i.e., the parents, donor, and physician. The status of the offspring has been of secondary concern. Now that there are a significant number of donor offspring reaching their middle years, they can contribute an important perspective on how donor insemination impacts their lives.

Most research on the experience of donor offspring has involved interviews with the parents of young children. I find this research limited for two reasons. Parents who have struggled to have children might find it difficult to be unbiased as to their children's experience. It might be important for their own psyche to see their children's experience biased toward a more positive light. Donor offspring "appear often to be 'special' children from the very beginning, just as are children who were born very premature" (Stotland, 1990, p. 164). This type of research is really about the parents' perceptions, not the offsprings' experience.

Also, research on young children is limited in that it does not allow a foretelling of what that person's experience will be as they age, as they are adolescents or adults. We can not draw conclusions about what their life experience will be.

As donor offspring age and more become known as donor offspring privately and publicly, we have an opportunity to research their experience as adolescents and as adults. The donor offspring in this study all did not know their status as donor offspring until they were adults. They were informed between the ages of 18 and 47.

It will also be important to study the experience of offspring who grow up knowing their status as donor offspring. The Sperm Bank of California has an open program of donor insemination, where the donor is willing to meet the offspring one time when they reach eighteen years of age. It will be very important to see what the experience of these offspring are.

Comparisons can be made between the experiences of offspring and families who keep donor insemination secret versus those who make it an open disclosure. Secrecy has historically been an important aspect of donor insemination, but its value is being seriously questioned.

For mental health practitioners, the effects of family secrets on parent-to-parent and parent-to-child relationships are considered destructive. Nowhere in the psychological literature is there any evidence to justify secrets, nor are there any studies that indicate the value of secrets. There is a great deal of evidence to the contrary. Our study corroborated this, and led us to the understanding of the need for openness and honesty. (Baran & Pannor, 1993, xii)

By comparing the experience of families with and without secrecy, the impact of secrecy can be more clearly distinguished from other dynamics in families.

It will be important to study the experience of openness in donor insemination for the sperm donor as well. There are fears and claims among those doing donor insemination that if it becomes an open system, then people will not want to be donors and donor insemination as a practice will be in jeopardy. Studying open donors experiences will help determine if this perception is accurate or not.

There are few studies directly seeking the experience of older donor offspring. Geithner (1988) was the first to interview adult donor offspring about their experiences. Her results showed the importance of access to medical information, educating and counseling parents about the implications of donor insemination, and advising parents to tell donor offspring of their origins. Turner (1999) focused on the identity experiences of adult donor offspring. Her results showed mistrust in families where donor offspring grew up not knowing their conception status, a sense of knowing there was secrecy in the family, a feeling of not belonging in the family, imbalance in family dynamics, a need to know their origins and search for their donor, and a need to talk to someone who values and respects their identities as donor offspring. These two studies, as well as Baran and Pannor all indicate a need for openness in donor insemination families.

My study focused on adult donor offspring confronting the reality of their status as donor offspring. The themes which were relevant for donor offspring included: regret, anger, a feeling of injustice regarding secrecy, feeling different from other people and experiencing discomfort telling others due to lack of understanding by others of their experience, doubt about paternity and a feeling of not fitting in their families, identity confusion, searching for the sperm donor and need for ancestral connection, searching for half-siblings and feeling a connection with them, concern about unknown inherited medical conditions for themselves and future generations, feeling alone and needing contact and support, finding support and similarities with adoptees, experiencing an array of strong positive and negative feelings, wanting to normalize and accept the reality of their status, developing beliefs that knowledge of their genetic and medical history are a birthright, finding a sense of purpose, and speaking out about their experience as a donor offspring. These results validated and expanded upon Geithner, Baran and Pannor, and Turner's conclusions.

Any of the themes in the experience of donor offspring could be studied more in depth. One area in particular which I would like to see more research on is the experience of abandonment for donor offspring. For adoptees, feeling abandoned by birthparents is a major part of their experience. For donor offspring, it is less clear. One of my co-researchers states "I didn't feel abandoned." Personally, in my experience, I did feel a sense of abandonment. Turner (1999) concludes that donor offspring "perceived a sense of abandonment by their donor fathers and the medical profession."

When donor offspring didn't know their genetic history, they experienced a feeling of non-existence or of not being whole. They gave visual descriptions of feeling split in half. It is important to study more about identity issues and feelings of not being a whole person. By comparing the experiences of donor offspring who know their true identity growing up versus those who are raised in secrecy, one would be able to separate out whether the identity issues are related to the effects of secrecy on family dynamics or to the fact of being a donor offspring and being separated from a genetic parent.

In society, there has been a severe lack of knowledge about the practice and psychological implications of donor insemination. Donor offspring have suffered because of a lack of understanding from other people as to what their experience is all about. As many topics become more open in our culture so, too, does donor insemination. There are many discussions in the media now about unraveling the genetic code, infertility issues, cloning, and ethical implications of genetic issues. The newer procedures and research have become spotlighted. Since donor insemination is not new, it has been more in the background of these discussions. It will be important for the ethical implications of all of these practices, including donor insemination, to be taken into serious consideration.

Ethical implications lead to the need for political regulation of these practices. There is a need for politicians to review the psychological and ethical impact of all of these practices and set policy to protect individuals. Historically, there has not been regulation of donor insemination practices. In the United States, the American Society for Reproductive Medicine has developed voluntary guidelines for donor insemination, as well as other reproductive technologies. I question if a group of individuals can fairly regulate themselves. Can fertility physicians, who have economic incentives and a powerful lobbying force, be trusted to consider what is best psychologically for parents and offspring? Donor families, donor offspring, and donors should be taken into consideration when determining policies regarding donor insemination. I feel there needs to be regulation outside of the system to ensure that practices are done in the best interest of those whose lives are impacted.

Byrne (1988) states that Senator Al Gore asked the Food and Drug Administration to require that physicians and sperm banks screen semen for HIV antibodies. Also at that time he was writing a bill to establish a national data bank for medical and genetic histories of anonymous donors so that children born through artificial insemination will have access to the data (p. 895). These protections should be followed through within the government structure in order to have assurance of compliance.

As more is understood about the experience of donor insemination, secrecy versus openness, relationships in the families, and other psychological components related to donor insemination, this information can be applied clinically by mental health practitioners. More understanding can be brought to working with individuals and families involved in donor insemination. For people involved with donor insemination, the more acceptance of the situation and of offspring for being who they are, including characteristics which come from the mother, social father, and genetic father, the more acceptance the offspring will have of themselves and the healthier relationships will be. New knowledge about the psychological implications related to donor offspring and relationships in donor families can be incorporated into the education of medical and mental health practitioners so they can use this clinically.

Another important aspect of clinical applications is bringing new knowledge and understanding of donor insemination into the public arena. The general public is largely uninformed about the prevalence and reality of the donor conception experience. Donor offspring express difficulty talking to others because of this lack of understanding and disbelief about donor insemination. Personally, I had a forensics police detective tell me that he didn't believe the reason I wanted to find out about laboratories that do DNA testing was because I was a donor offspring. He said he had never heard of it before. There must be a different reason I wanted this information. That was in 1993. Clinicians can help increase public awareness, as well as apply understanding of donor insemination issues in their own practices.

In making decisions about whether and how to use donor insemination in their families, people will benefit from more knowledge and understanding of implications of donor insemination. They can learn more about this by reading current literature, and talking with physicians and mental health clinicians, in order to make informed decisions about donor insemination in their own lives. The American Society for Reproductive Medicine guidelines for recipients of donor insemination state: "The decision to proceed with donor insemination is emotionally complex. Patients may benefit from psychologic counseling to aid in this decision." (American Society for Reproductive Medicine, 2000, p. 2).

In conclusion, very little research has been done regarding psychological implications of donor insemination from the perspective of donor offspring. There is a need for more research, especially of the experiences of donor offspring during adolescence and adulthood, comparing the effects of secrecy versus openness, and considering identity/existential concerns. Donor offspring feel a need for openness in donor insemination practices, and they believe that knowledge of genetic heritage is a birthright. More understanding of the issues by physicians, mental health practitioners, and the public at large, and legislation protecting the rights of donor offspring is imperative. Learning from the experience of participants of donor insemination can be instrumental as other reproductive technologies expand.

REFERENCES

Achilles, R.G. (1987). The social meanings of biological ties: A study of participants in artificial insemination by donor. Ottawa, Canada: National Library of Canada. Unpublished doctoral dissertation, University of Toronto.

Adler, G., & Myerson, P.G. (1991). Confrontation in psychotherapy. Northvale, NJ: Jason Aronson.

American Psychological Association. (1992). Ethical principles of psychologists and code of conduct. American Psychologist, 47(12), 1597-1161.

American Society for Reproductive Medicine. (2000). Guidelines for gamete and embryo donation. Birmingham, AL: American Society for Reproductive Medicine.

Baran, A., & Pannor, R. (1993). Lethal secrets: The psychology of donor insemination problems and solutions. New York: Amistad.

Berenson, B.G., & Mitchell, K.M. (1974). Confrontation for better or worse! Amherst, MA: Human Resource Development Press.

Berger, D.M. (1982). Psychological aspects of donor insemination. International Journal of Psychiatry Medicine, 12(1), 49-57.

Blyth, E., Crawshaw, M., & Speirs, J. (Eds.). (1998). Truth and the child 10 years on: Information exchange in donor assisted conception. Birmingham, Great Britain: British Association of Social Workers.

Botsford, J.S. (2000, Spring). A personal story of blood and belonging. DC Network News, (15), 10-11.

Briggs, B. (1997, November 9). Family secrets. <u>Denver Post,</u> p. D1.

Brown, M.R. (1994, March 7). Whose eyes are these, whose nose? <u>Newsweek, 123</u>(10), 12.

Burleigh, N. (1999, March). Are you my father? <u>Redbook, 192</u>(5), 108-111.

Byrne, G. (1988, August 19). Artificial insemination report prompts call for regulation. (Office of Technology Assessment report). <u>Science, 241</u>, 895.

Chan, R.W., Raboy, B., & Patterson, C.J. (1998, April). Psychosocial adjustment among children conceived via donor insemination by lesbian and heterosexual mothers. <u>Child Development, 69</u>(2), 443-457.

(1998, September 28). The children of sperm donors: Pressure grows to identify anonymous fathers. <u>Maclean's, 111</u>(39), 56.

Cobb, N. (1992, September 10). Who is my donor dad? <u>Boston Globe,</u> p. 85.

Cook, T., & Reichardt, C. (Eds.). (1979). <u>Qualitative and quantitative methods in evaluation research.</u> Beverly Hills, CA: Sage.

Cordray, B. (1999/2000, Winter). An open letter to the HFEA (Human Fertilisation and Embryology Act). <u>DI Network News, 14</u>, 3-5.

Corsini, R.J. (1999). <u>The dictionary of psychology.</u> Philadelphia: Brunner/Mazel.

Daniels, K.R., & Haimes, E. (Eds.). (1998). <u>Donor insemination: International social science perspectives.</u> New York: Cambridge University Press.

Donor Conception Support Group of Australia. (Ed.). (1997). <u>Let the offspring speak: Discussions on donor conception.</u> New South Wales, Australia: Donor Conception Support Group of Australia.

Franz, S. (2000). Sperm, secrets, and information-sharing. Unpublished journal article.

Geithner, C.S. (1988). The secret of artificial insemination by donor: The offsprings experience: A research project based upon an independent investigation. (Thesis, Smith College School for Social Work).

Giorgi, A., Fischer, W., & Von Eckartsberg, R. (1971). Duquesne Studies in Phenomenological Psychology: Vol. I. Pittsburgh: Duquesne University Press.

Golombok, S., Murray, C., Brinsen, P., & Abdalla H. (1999). Social versus biological parenting: Family functioning and the socioemotional development of children conceived by egg or sperm donation. Journal of Child Psychology & Psychiatry & Allied Disciplines, 40(4), 519-527.

Karlsson, G. (1993). Psychological qualitative research from a phenomenological perspective. Sweden: Graphic Systems AB.

Kinross, L. (1992, July 25). Breaking the silence on donor insemination. Toronto Star.

Kovacs, G.T., Mushin, D., Kane, H., & Baker, H.W.G. (1993). A controlled study of the psycho-social development of children conceived following insemination with donor semen. Human Reproduction, 8(5), 788-790.

Landsberg, M. (2000, April 2). Children need to know sperm donors. The Toronto Star, p. A2.

Leeton, J., & Backwell, J. (1982). A preliminary psychosocial follow-up of parents and their children conceived by artificial insemination by donor (AID). Clinical Reproductive Fertility, 1(4), 307-310.

Moustakas, C. (1994). Phenomenological research methods. Thousand Oaks, CA: Sage.

Noble, E. (1987). Having your baby by donor insemination: A complete resource guide. Boston: Houghton Mifflin.

Norton, C. (2000, April 24). 'Faceless fathers' may be identified. The Independent, London, Great Britain.

NZPA. (2000, June 14). Register of 'genetic parents' urged. New Zealand News from The Press.

O'Brien, K. (1996). Artificial insemination by donor: The voice of the unborn child. Unpublished master's thesis, Metropolitan State College of Denver.

Orenstein, P. (1995, June 18). Looking for a donor to call dad. The New York Times Magazine, p. 28.

Patton, M. (1975). Alternative evaluation research paradigm. Grand Forks, ND: University of North Dakota Press.

Rogers, C.R. (1980). A way of being. Boston: Houghton Mifflin.

Rubin, S. (1995, January 15). Family secrets. San Francisco Chronicle, p. S1.

Schellen, A.M.C.M. (1957). Artificial insemination in the human. Amsterdam: Elsevier Publishing Company.

Sokoloff, B.Z. (1987). Alternative methods of reproduction. Effects on the child. Clinical Pediatrics, 26(1), 11-17.

Stotland, N. (Ed.). (1990). Psychiatric aspects of reproductive technology. Washington, DC: American Psychiatric Press.

Topp, K. (1993). Positive reflections: Growing up as a DI child. The Canadian Journal of Human Sexuality, 2(3).

Turner, A. (1999, December). What does it mean to be a donor offspring? The identity experiences of adults conceived by donor insemination and implications for counselling and therapy. (Research summary received from author, unnumbered). Surrey, UK: University of Surrey, Department of Psychology, School of Human Sciences.

Valle, R. (Ed.). (1998). <u>Phenomenological inquiry in psychology: Existential and transpersonal dimensions.</u> New York: Plenum Press.

Verny, T.R. (1994). The stork in the lab: Biological, psychological, ethical, social and legal aspects of third party conceptions. <u>Pre- & Peri-Natal Psychology Journal, 9</u>(1), 57-84.

White, C. (1998). Banking on interest. <u>British Medical Journal, 317</u>(7158), 607.

APPENDIX A
RELATED RESOURCES

Abrams, T. (1994, March). My test-tube daddy. <u>Washingtonian,</u> <u>29</u>(6), 44.

Achilles, R.G. (1992). <u>Donor insemination: An overview.</u> Ottawa, CANADA: Royal Commission on New Reproductive Technologies.

Achilles, R.G. (1993). Protection from what? The secret life of donor insemination. <u>Politics and the Life Sciences, 12</u>(2), 171-172.

Adair, V.A., & Purdie, A. (1996). Donor insemination programmes with personal donors: issues of secrecy. <u>Human Reproduction, 11</u>(11), 2558-2563.

Adair, V., & Sutherland, C. (1991). <u>Donor insemination: Issues of</u> <u>secrecy and related areas: A selective annotated bibliography.</u> Fertility Associates.

All in a day's work, Dr. Amanda Turner, Donor insemination counselling pshycologist. (2001, October 22). <u>The Eveing Standard</u> (London, England), p. 13.

American Fertility Society. (1993). Guidelines for gamete donation: 1993. <u>Fertility and Sterility, 59</u> (Suppl. 1), 1S-9S.

American Fertility Society. (1990). New guidelines for the use of semen donor insemination, 1990. <u>Fertility and Sterility, 53</u> (Suppl.).

American Fertility Society. (1986). New guidelines for the use of semen donor insemination, 1986. <u>Fertility and Sterility, 46</u> (Suppl. 2).

American Fertility Society. (1991). Revision of guidelines for the use of semen donor insemination: 1991. Fertility and Sterility, 56(3), 396.

American Society for Reproductive Medicine. (2006, November). 2006 Guidelines for gamete and embryo donation. Fertility and Sterility, 86 (Suppl 4), S38-S50.

American Society for Reproductive Medicine, Ethics Committee. (1997). Ethical considerations of assisted reproductive technologies. Fertility and Sterility, 67 (Suppl. 1), i-iii,1S-9S.

American Society for Reproductive Medicine. (1998). Guidelines for gamete and embryo donation. Fertility and Sterility, 70 (Suppl. 3), 1S-13S.

American Society for Reproductive Medicine. (2004, March). Informing offspring of their conception by gamete donation. Fertility and Sterility, 81, 527-531.

American Society for Reproductive Medicine. (2006, November). Revised minimum standards for practices offering assisted reproductive technologies. Fertility and Sterility, 86 (Suppl 4), S53-S56.

Amuzu, B., Laxova, R., & Shapiro, S.S. (1990). Pregnancy outcome, health of children, and family adjustment after donor insemination. Obstetrics and Gynecology, 75(6), 899-905.

Annas, G.J. (1989). The ethics of genetic control: ending reproductive roulette. The Journal of the American Medical Association, 261(3), 453. (book review)

Anonymous. (1999, October 14). Origin unknown: Sperm donors want to keep it that way. The Guardian. (available in the DI Network News, Winter 1999/2000)

Ansorge, R. (1998, November 3). Book shares stories of adults who had children in unconventional ways. Knight-Ridder/Tribune News Service, p. K7323.

Appleton, T. (1991). Donor insemination: A guide for patients. Cambridge, MA: Infertility Support Couselling.

Appleton, T. (1991). The use of donor sperm: A guide for patients. Cambridge, MA: Infertility Support Couselling.

Askin, J., & Davis, M. (1992). Search: A handbook for adoptees and birthparents (2nd ed.). Phoenix, AR: Oryx Press.

Audi, T. (2006, June 15). From 'donor 48QAH' to dad. USA Today, p. 07D.

Back, K.W., & Snowden, R. (1988). The anonymity of the gamete donor and Psychological and ethical concerns in new reproductive technologies. Journal of Psychosomatic Obstetrics & Gynaecology, 9(3). 191-198. (Special Issue).

Baker, D.J., & Paterson, M.A. (1995). Marketed sperm: Use and regulation in the United States. Fertility and Sterility, 63(5), 947-952.

Barratt, C.L.R., & Cooke, I.D. (Eds.). (1993). Donor insemination. Cambridge, NY: Cambridge University Press.

Barratt, C.L.R., & Matson, P.L., Holt, W. (1993). British Andrology Society guidelines for the screening of semen donors for donor insemination. Human Reproduction, 8(9), 1521.

Barrett, H. (1989, June). Anything for a baby. Redbook, 173(2), 64.

Barrett, S.E. (1997). Children of lesbian parents: The what, when and how of talking about donor identity. Women & Therapy, 20(2), 43-55.

Bartholet, E. (1993). Family bonds: Adoption and the politics of parenting. Boston: Houghton Mifflin.

BBC. (1999, August 23). Test tube dads: The inside story. Arts and Entertainment T.V. (interviews with Xytex sperm donors, and meeting between donor and offspring)

Becker, G. (1990). Healing the infertile family: Strengthening your relationship in the search for parenthood. Berkeley, CA: University of California Press.

Being a child of donor insemination. (2002, June 1). British Medical Journal, 324(7349), 1339.

Belmont, M.F.L. (1979/80). Attitudes and knowledges of maternity nurses concerning artificial insemination by donor. Unpublished doctoral dissertation, Teacher's College, Columbia University, New York.

Bendvold, E., Moe, N., & Skjaeraasen, J. (1990). Social conditions of children born after artificial insemination by donor. Scandinavian Journal of Social Medicine, 18(3), 203-206.

Bennett, B., & Tomossy, G.F (2006, May 11). Globalization and health: Challenges for health law and bioethics (International Library of Ethics, Law, and the New Medicine). The Netherlands: Springer.

Bennett, V. (1998, November 6). The unknown fathers. (Rights of children born following donor insemination to trace fathers). The Times, p. 23.

Berger, D.M. (1980). Infertility. A psychiatrist's perspective. Canadian Journal of Psychiatry, 25(7), 553-559.

Berger, D.M., Eisen, A., Shuber, J., & Doody, K.F. (1986). Psychological patterns in donor insemination couples. Canadian Journal of Psychiatry, 31(9), 818-823.

Bernstein, A.C. (1994). Flight of the stork: What children think (and when) about sex and family building. Indianapolis, IN: Perspectives Press.

Bernthal, N. (1990). Lost and found: The experience of becoming an adoptive mother to a foreign-born child. (Doctoral Dissertation, The Union Institute, 1990). Dissertation Abstracts International, 51(06), 3120B.

Bielawska-Batorowicz, E. (1994). Artificial insemination by donor— An investigation of recipient couples' viewpoints. Journal of Reproductive and Infant Psychology, 12(2), 123.

Blaser, A., Maloigne-Katz, B., & Gigon, U. (1988). Effect of artificial insemination with donor semen on the psyche of the husband. Psychotherapy and Psychosomatics, 49(1), 17-21.

Blizzard, J. (1977). Blizzard and the holy ghost: Artificial insemination: A personal account. London: Peter Owen.

Blum, H.P. (1996). The secret seed of hatred in a delinquent adolescent. Madison, CT: International Universities Press.

Blyth, E. (1998). Donor assisted conception and donor offspring rights to genetic origins information. The International Journal of Children's Rights, 6(3), 237-253.

Blyth, E. (1999, Spring). Secrets and lies: Barriers to the exchange of genetic origins information following donor assisted conception. Adoption & Fostering Journal, 23(1), 49-58.

Blyth, E., Crawshaw, M., Haase, J., & Speirs, J. (2001, November). The implications of adoption for donor offspring following donor-assisted conception. Child & Family Social Work, 6(4), 295-304.

Blyth, E., & Hunt, J. (1998, November). Sharing genetic origins information in donor assisted conception: Views from licensed centres on HFEA donor information form (91) 4. Human Reproduction, 13(11), 3274-3277.

Blyth, E., & Landau, R. (2004, December). Third party assisted conception across cultures: Social, legal and ethical perspective. London, England and New York, NY: Jessica Kingsley Publishers.

Boggan, S. (2002, July 27). Children born of sperm donors win right to take on Government. The Independent, p. 9.

Bolton, V., Golombok, S., Cook, R., Bish, A., & Rust, J. (1991). A comparative study of attitudes towards donor insemination and egg donation in recipients, potential donors and the public. Journal of Psychosomatic Obstetrics and Gynaecology, 12(3), 217-228.

Brand, H.J. (1987). Complexity of motivation for artificial insemination by donor. Psychol Rep, 60(3 Pt 1), 951-955.

Brewaeys, A. (1996). Donor insemination, the impact on family and child development. Journal of Psychosomatic Obstetrics and Gynaecology, 17(1), 1-13.

Brewaeys, A. (2001, February). Review: Parent-child relationships and child development in donor insemination families. Human Reproduction Update, 7(1), 38-46.

Brewaeys, A., Ponjaert-Kristoffersen, I., Van Steirteghem, A.C., & Devroey, P. (1993). Children from anonymous donors: an inquiry into homosexual and heterosexual parents' attitudes. Journal of Psychosomatic Obstetrics and Gynaecology, 14(Suppl.), 23-35.

Brewaeys, A., Golombok, S., Naaktgeboren, N., & De Bruyn, J.K. (1997). Donor insemination: Dutch parents' opinions about confidentiality and donor anonymity and the emotional adjustment of their children. Human Reproduction, 12(7), 1591-1597.

Britain to let test-tube children trace donors. (1999, July 26). The Seattle Times, p. A3.

British Andrology Society guidelines for the screening of semen donors for donor insemination. (1999). Human Reproduction, 14(7), 1823.

Brits to get right to trace genetics. (1999, July 26). Tulsa World, p. 4.

Brody, L. (1998, November 3). The facts of life for technology's children: Old answers won't do for miracle kids. Knight-Ridder/Tribune News Service, p. K7328.

Brodzinsky, D.M., Schechter, M.D., & Henig, R.M. (1992). Being adopted: The lifelong search for self. New York: Anchor Books.

Brotherton, J. (1990). Artificial insemination with fresh donor semen. Archives of Andrology, 25(2), 173.

Bruce, N., Mitchell, A., & Priestley K. (1988). Truth and the child: A contribution to the debate on the Warnock report. Edinburgh: Family Care.

Burns, L.H. (1999). Genetics and infertility: Psychosocial issues in reproductive counseling. Families, Systems & Health, 17(1), 87.

Burns, L.H. (1999). Infertility counseling: A comprehensive handbook for clinicians. Pearl River, NY: Parthenon Publishing Group.

Callahan, S. (1994, November 18). Kinship is forever. Commonweal, 121(20), 5.

Callahan, S. (1987, April 24). Lovemaking & babymaking. Commonweal, 114, 233-239.

Call to identify sperm donor in human rights test case. (2000, September 11). The Guardian, p. 1.

Callus, T. (2004, July). Tempered Hope? A qualified right to know one's genetic origin: Odievre v France. Modern Law Review, 67(4), 658-669.

Capron, A.M. (1998, September). Too many parents. The Hastings Center Report, p. 22.

Carp, E.W. (2000, April 7). Family matters: Secrecy and disclosure in the history of adoption. USA: First Harvard University Press.

Carp, E.W. (1998). Secrecy and disclosure in the history of adoption. Cambridge, MA: Harvard University Press.

Carr, E.K., Friedman, T., Lannon, B., & Sharp, P.C. (1990). The study of psychological factors in couples receiving artificial insemination by donor: A discussion of methodological difficulties. Journal of Advanced Nursing, 15(8), 906-910.

Carter, C.O. (1983). Developments in human reproduction and their eugenic, ethical implications: Proceedings of the nineteenth annual symposium of the Eugenics Society, London 1982. Eugenics Society, London, England: Academic Press.

Children born by donated sperm 'liable to suffer identity crisis' researchers claim. (2000, August 31). The Guardian, p. 9.

The children of sperm donors: Pressure grows to identify anonymous fathers. (1998, September 28). Maclean's, 111(39), 56.

Chisholm, P. (1999, December 6). For infertile couples, heartache and hope: Despite the discomforts and the long odds, would-be parents turn to doctors and donors to deliver what nature could not. Maclean's, p. 58.

Clamar, A.J. (1984). Artificial insemination by donor: The anonymous pregnancy. American Journal of Forensic Psychology, 2(1), 27-37.

Clamar, A. (1980). Psychological implications of donor insemination. American Journal of Psychoanalysis, 40(2), 173-177.

Clark, R.A. (1992). Intramarital illegitimacy. Medicine & Law, 11(3-4), 309-312.

Clark, V., & Titchen, A. (1997, April 27). Adam's invisible dad. The Observer, p. 11.

Clarke, G.N., Bourne, H., Hill, P., & Johnston, W.I.H. (1997). Artificial insemination and in-vitro fertilization using donor spermatozoa: A report on 15 years of experience. Human Reproduction, 12(4), 722.

Clayton, C.E., & Kovacs, G.T. (1982). AID offspring: Initial follow-up study of 50 couples. Medical Journal of Australia, 1(8), 338-339.

Clement, J.L. (1993). Psycho-sociological profile of a series of 850 sperm donors. Contraception, Fertilite, Sexualite, 21(6), 498-500.

Cohen, S.R. (2004, October). The invisible man. Artificial insemination by donor and the legislation on donor anonymity: A review. Journal of Family Planning and Reproductive Health Care, 30(4), 270-273.

Connolly, K.J., Edelmann, R.J., Cooke, I.D., & Robson, J. (1992). The impact of infertility on psychological functioning. Journal of Psychosomatic Research, 36(5), 459-468.

Cook, R.E. (1990/1). Psychological functioning in couples undergoing in vitro fertilisation (IVF) or donor insemination (DI) treatment for infertility. Unpublished doctoral dissertation, The City University, London, UK.

Cook, R., Golombok, S., Bish A., & Murray, C. (1995). Disclosure of donor insemination: Parental attitudes. American Journal of Orthopsychiatry, 65(4), 549-559.

Cook, R., Parsons, J., Mason, B., & Golombok, S. (1989). Emotional, marital and sexual functioning in patients embarking upon IVF and AID treatment for infertility (special issue). Journal of Reproductive & Infant Psychology, 7(2), 87-93.

Cooke, I. (1993). Secrecy, openness, and DI in the UK. Politics and the Life Sciences, p. 176-177.

Cooper, S. (1998). Choosing assisted reproduction: Social, emotional & ethical considerations. Indianapolis, IN: Perspectives Press.

Cooper, S.L., & Glazer, E.S. (1994). Beyond infertility: The new paths to parenthood. New York: Lexington Books.

Cordray, B. The need for a sense of self-identity. (available from the Infertility Network)

Corson, S.L., & Mechanick-Braverman, A. (1998). Why we believe there should be a gamete registry. Fertility and Sterility, 69(5), 809-811.

Cox, D.N., & Reading, A.E. (1983). Personality profiles of women attending an artificial insemination by donor clinic. Personality & Individual Differences, 4(2), 213-214.

Crawshaw, M. (2002). Lessons from a recent adoption study to identify some of the service needs of, and issues for, donor offspring wanting to know about their donors. Human Fertility, 5(1), 6-12.

Crawshaw, M.A., Blyth, E.D., & Daniels, K.D. (2007, April). Past semen donors' views about the use of a voluntary contact register. Reproductive BioMedicine Online, 14(4), 411-417.

Creighton, P. (1977). Artificial insemination by donor: A study of ethics, medicine, and law in our technological society. Toronto: Anglican Book Centre.

Cryogenics Laboratories, Inc. (1995). Choosing parenthood through donor insemination. Roseville, MN: Cryogenic Laboratories. (videocassette).

Czyba, J.C., & Chevret, M. (1979). Psychological reactions of couples to artificial insemination with donor sperm. International Journal of Fertility, 24(4), 240-245.

Dad is not my natural father: Dear Deidre. (2000, November 25). The Sun, p. 43.

Daly, K., & Sobol, M. (1992, Oct.). Highlights from adoption as an alternative for infertile couples: Prospects and trends. Excerpts from a study prepared for The Royal Commission on the New Reproductive Technologies.

Danesh-Meyer, H.V., Gillett, W.R., & Daniels, K.R. (1993). Withdrawal from a donor insemination programme. The Australian and New Zealand Journal of Obstetrics & Gynaecology, 33(2), 187-189.

Daniels, K.R. (1994). Adoption and donor insemination: Factors influencing couples' choices. Child Welfare, 73(1), 5-14.

Daniels, K.R. (1988). Artificial insemination using donor semen and the issue of secrecy: The views of donors and recipient couples. Social Science and Medicine, 27(4), 377-383.

Daniels, K.R. (1990). Attitudes to donor insemination and in vitro fertilization—A community perspective. Social Work and Society, 1(1), 4-10.

Daniels, K.R. (1997). The controversy regarding privacy versus disclosure among patients using donor gametes in assisted reproductive technology. Journal of Assisted Reproductive Genetics, 14(7), 373-375.

Daniels, K. (2007, February). Donor gametes: Anonymous or identified? Best Practice & Research Clinical Obstetrics &Gynaecology, 21(1), 113.

Daniels, K.R. (1996). Gamete donation and its impact on relationships. Western Australia Roproductive Technology Council Annual Report, Appendix 4, pp. ii—xi.

Daniels, K.R. (1995). Information sharing in donor insemination: A conflict of rights and needs. Cambridge Quarterly of Healthcare Ethics, 4, 217-224.

Daniels, K.R. (1997). Information sharing in semen donation: The views of donors. Social Science & Medicine, 44(5), 673-680.

Daniels, K. (2005, December). Is blood really thicker than water? Assisted reproduction and its impact on our thinking about family. Journal of Psychosomatic Obstetrics & Gynecology, 26(4), 265-270.

Daniels, K.R. (1993). Moving towards openness in donor insemination: Variations on a theme. Politics and the Life Sciences, 12(2), 200-203.

Daniels, K.R. (1986). New birth technologies: A social work approach to researching the psychosocial factors. Social Work Health Care, 11(4), 49-60.

Daniels, K.R. (1986). Psychosocial issues associated with being a semen donor. Clinical Reproduction and Fertility, 4(5), 341-351.

Daniels, K.R. (Ed.). (1998). Psychosocial perspectives on donor insemination : International social science perspectives. New York: Cambridge University Press.

Daniels, K.R. (1989). Semen donors: Their motivations and attitudes to their offspring. Journal of Reproductive and Infant Psychology, 7, 121-127.

Daniels, K. (2001, September). Sharing information with donor insemination offspring. Human Reproduction, 16(9), 1792-1796.

Daniels, K.R. (1994). The Swedish Insemination Act and its impact. Australia New Zealand Journal of Obstetrics and Gynecology, 34(4), 437-439.

Daniels, K., Blyth, E., Crawshaw, M., & Curson, R. (2005, June 1). Short Communication: Previous semen donors and their views regarding the sharing of information with offspring. Human Reproduction, 20(6), 1670-1675.

Daniels, K.R., & Fairweather, J.R. (1983). Artificial insemination by donor: A bibliography. Christchurch, NZ: Social Work Unit, Department of Sociology, University of Canterbury.

Daniels, K.R., Gillett, W.R., & Herbison, G.P. (1996). Successful donor insemination and its impact on recipients. Journal of Psychosomatic Obstetrics and Gynaecology, 17(3), 129-134.

Daniels, K., & Haimes, E. (1998, May 28). Donor insemination: International social science perspectives. Cambridge, United Kingdom and New York, NY: Cambridge University Press.

Daniels, K., Lalos, A., Gottlieb, C., & Lalos, O. (2005, March). Semen providers and their three families. Journal of Psychosomatic Obstetrics & Gynecology, 26(1), 15-22.

Daniels, K., & Lalos, O. (1995). The Swedish insemination act and the availability of donors. Human Reproduction, 10(7), 1871-1874.

Daniels, K.R., & Lewis, G.M. (1996). Donor insemination: The gifting and selling of semen. Social Science & Medicine, 42(11), 1521-1536.

Daniels, K.R., & Lewis, G.M. (1996). Openness of information in the use of donor gametes: Developments in New Zealand. Journal of Reproductive & Infant Psychology, 14(1), 57-68.

Daniels, K.R., Lewis, G.M., & Gillett, W. (1995). Telling donor insemination offspring about their conception: The nature of couples' decision-making. Social Science & Medicine, 40(9), 1213-1220.

Daniels, K., & Meadows, L. (2006, June). Sharing information with adults conceived as a result of donor insemination. Human Fertility, 9(2), 93-99.

Daniels, K., & Taylor, K. (1993). Secrecy and openness in donor insemination. Politics and the Life Sciences, 12(2), 155-170.

David, D., Soule, M., Mayaux, M.J., Guimard-Moscato, M.L., Czyglik, F., Levy, A., Cahen, F., Bissery, J., Noel, J., & Schwartz, D. (1988). Donor artificial insemination. Psychological survey of 830 couples. Journal of Gynecologie, Obstetrique et Biologie de la Reproduction, 17(1), 67-74.

Deech, R. (1998, February 6). Letter: Internet dads. The Guardian, p. O18.

Deech, R. (1996). A patient's guide to donor insemination and in-vitro fertilization clinics. Human Reproduction, 11(7), 1363.

Desmond, C. (1999, July 13). Last night's TV: Seeds of doubt. The Guardian, p. T022.

DiGiantomasso, F. (1983). Proceedings of the conference: Ethical implications in the use of donor sperm, eggs and embryos in the treatment of human infertility. Clayton, Victoria: Centre for Human Bioethics, Monash University.

DI Network. What shall we tell the children? The Globe and Mail. (available from the Infertility Network)

Disclosure hope for sperm donor offspring. (2002, July 27). The Guardian, p. 7.

Donor anonymity in artificial insemination: Is it still necessary? (1993). Columbia Journal of Law and Social Problems, 27(1), 151.

'Donor' children get the right to know. (2001, November 16). The Times, p. 2.

Donor insemination: The emotional effects. (1993, May/June). Reprint from The Parkway Fertility Report.

Donor offspring find their missing links. (2005, June 2). The Times, p. 16.

Dresser, R. (2000, November 1). Regulating Assisted Reproduction. The Hastings Center Report, 30(6), 26.

Drews, S.E. (1997). The experience of being wounded with individuals adopted at birth. Unpublished master's thesis, Center for Humanistic Studies, Detroit, MI.

Dunnington, R.M., & Estok, P.J. (1991). Potential psychological attachments formed by donors involved in fertility technology-another side to infertility. Nurse Practitioner, 16(11), 41-48.

Durna, E.M., Bebe, J., Leader, L.R., Steigrad, S.J., & Garrett, D.G. (1995). Donor insemination: Effects on parents. Medical Journal of Australia, 163(5), 248-251.

Durna, E.M., Bebe, J., Steigrad, S.J., Leader, L.R., & Garrett, D.G. (1997). Donor insemination: Attitudes of parents towards disclosure. Medical Journal of Australia, 167(5), 256-259.

Dyer, C. (2000, September 16). Offspring from artificial insemination demand fathers' details. British Medical Journal, 321(7262), 654.

Dyer, C. (2002, May 25). Pressure increases on government to remove anonymity from sperm donors. British Medical Journal, 324(7348), 1237.

Ebtehaj, F., Lindley, B., & Richards, M. (2006, September). Kinship Matters. Portland, Oregon: Hart Publishing.

Edelmann, R.J. (1996). Psychological factors relating to semen donation: A comment. Human Reproduction, 11(12), 2571-2572.

Ehlert, B. (1992, March 11). Do you tell the kids? Chicago Tribune, p. 7.

Ehrensaft, D. (2000, October 15). Alternatives to the stork: Fatherhood fantasies in donor insemination families. Studies in Gender and Sexuality, 1(4), 371-397.

Emond, M. (1998). Why not donate sperm? A study of potential donors. Evolution & Human Behavior, 19(5), 313-319.

Ending anonymity of sperm donors. (2004, January 28). The Times, p. 23.

Englert, Y. (1994). Artificial insemination with donor semen: Particular requests. Human Reproduction, 9(11), 1969.

LYNNE W SPENCER

English, C.B. (1977). The legal and public health aspects of donor artificial insemination. Unpublished master's thesis, University of Texas, Health Science Center at Houston, School of Public Health.

Ethical issues associated with the new reproductive technologies. (1997). New York: John Wiley & Sons.

Fader, S. (1993). Sperm Banking: A reproductive resource. CA: California Cryobank. (excerpt: History of Semen Banks. http://www.cryobank.com/history.html).

Farris, E.J., & Garrison, M. (1954). Emotional impact of successful donor insemination. A report on 38 couples. Obstetrics & Gynecology, 3(1), 19-20.

Fass, M. (2007, January 23). Man shares insemination responsibility. New York Law Journal.

Feast, J. (2003, February). Using and not losing the messages from the adoption experience for donor-assisted conception. Human Fertility, 6(1), 41-45.

Ferriman, A. (1994, February 15). What shall we tell our children? The Times, p. 4M.

Fidell, L.S., Marik, J., Donner, J.E., Jenkins-Burk, C., Koenigsberg, J., Magnussen, K., Morgan, C., & Ullman, J.B. (1989). Gender in transition: A new frontier. New York: Plenum Medical Book Company.

First contact: Sperm donor children. (2003, January 29). The Times, p. 7.

Ford, W.C. (2002). Male infertility: Tales of progress and frustration. Human Fertility, 5(1) S53-S60.

Foster-Fraser, K.L. (1990). Male donors' personality characteristics, parental relationships, and motivations to participate in artificial insemination. Unpublished doctoral dissertation, California School of Professional Psychology, Berkeley/Alameda.

Frank, D., & Vogel, M. (1988). The baby makers. New York: Carroll & Graf Publishers.

Franz, S. The sexual legacy of infertility: The separation of procreation and recreation. (available from the Infertility Network)

Freidrich, O. (1984, September 10). 'A legal, moral, social nightmare'; Society seeks to define the problems of the birth revolution. Time, 124, 54.

Frith, L. (2001, October). Beneath the rhetoric: The role of rights in the practice of non-anonymous gamete donation. Bioethics, 15(5-6), 473-484.

Frith, L. (2001, May). Gamete donation and anonymity. Human Reproduction, 16(5), 818-824.

Fulcher, M., Chan, R.W., Raboy, B., & Patterson, C.J. (2002). Contact with grandparents among children conceived via donor insemination by lesbian and heterosexual mothers. Parenting, 2(1), 61-76.

Gabel, S. (1988). Filling in the blanks: A guided look at growing up adopted. Fort Wayne, IN: Perspectives Press.

Gardner, M. (1998, October 28). Should children know donor parents? Christian Science Monitor, p. B5.

Gazvani, R., Hamilton, M., Simpson, S., & Templeton, A. (2002, November). New challenges for gamete donation programmes: Changes in guidelines are needed. Human Fertility, 5(4), 183-184.

Gera-Moglia, N.E. (1993). Siblings as gamete donors: An attitudinal survey of infertile couples and mental health professionals. Unpublished doctoral dissertation, Rutgers, The State University of New Jersey..

Gianelli, D.M. (1992). Benefits seen in regulating fertility medicine. American Medical News, 35(9), 3.

Gianelli, D.M. (1992). Fertility doctor's conviction fuels issue of self-policing. American Medical News, 35(12), 12.

Gillett, W.R., Daniels, K.R., & Herbison, G.P. (1996). Feelings of couples who have had a child by donor insemination: The degree of congruence. Journal of Psychosomatic Obstetrics and Gynaecology, 17(3), 135-142.

Glazer, E.S. (1998). The long-awaited stork: A guide to parenting after infertility. San Francisco: Jossey-Bass.

Golden, F., & Paul, A.M. (1999). Making over mom & dad: It's science and not the stork who often brings babies these days: In-vitro fertilization, donor insemination and other innovations have changed the way many women become pregnant. Psychology Today, 32(3), 36.

Gollancz, D. (2001, August). Donor insemination: A question of rights. Human Fertility, 4(3), 164-167.

Golombok, S. (1997). Parenting and secrecy issues related to children of assisted reproduction. Journal of Assisted Reproductive Genetics, 14(7), 375-378.

Golombok, S., Brewaeys, A., Giavazzi, M.T., Guerra, D., MacCallum, F., & Rust, J. (2002, March). Ethics and society. The European study of assisted reproduction families: The transition to adolescence. Human Reproduction, 17(3), 830-840.

Golombok, S., & Cook, R. (1994). A survey of semen donation: Phase I-The view of UK licensed centres. Human Reproduction, 9(5), 882-888.

Golombok, S., Cook, R., Bish, A., & Murray, C. (1995). Families created by the new reproductive technologies: Quality of parenting and social and emotional development of the children. Child Development, 66(2), 285-298. (Also found in Annual Progress in Child Psychiatry & Child Development, 1996, 529-550).

Golombok, S., Cook, R., Bish, A., & Murray, C. (1993). Quality of parenting in families created by the new reproductive technologies: A brief report of preliminary findings. Journal of Psychosomatic Obstetrics and Gynaecology, 14 (Suppl.), 17-22.

Golombok, S., Jadva, V., Lycett, E., Murray, C., & MacCallum, F. (2005, January 1). Families created by gamete donation: Follow-up at age 2. Human Reproduction, 20(1), 286-293.

Golombok, S., Lycett, E., MacCallum, F., & Jadva, V. (2004, September). Parenting infants conceived by gamete donation. Journal of Family Psychology, 18(3), 443-452.

Golombok, S., MacCallum, F., Goodman, E., & Rutter., M. (2002, May—June). Families with children conceived by donor insemination: A follow-up at age twelve. Child Development, 73(3), 952.

Golombok, S., & Rust, J. (1986). What about the children? Journal of Medical Ethics, 12(4), 182-186.

Golombok, S., & Tasker, F. (1994). Donor insemination for single heterosexual and lesbian women: Issues concerning the welfare of the child. Human Reproduction, 9(11), 1972.

Gordon, E., & Clo, K. (1992). Mommy did I grow in your tummy?— Where some babies come from. Santa Monica, CA: EM Greenbery Press. (My Story, by University Department of Obstetrics and Gynaecology. J.W. Northend, Ltd, 1991).

Gordon-Ceresky, D.L. (1995). Artificial insemination: Its effect on paternity and inheritance rights. The Connecticut Probate Law Journal, 9(2), 245-271.

Gottlieb, C., & Lalos, O. (2000, September). Ethics and society. Disclosure of donor insemination to the child: The impact of Swedish legislation on couples' attitudes. Human Reproduction, 15(9), 2052-2056.

Grand, C. (1997). New reproductive technologies: An overview of attitudes, opinions, acceptance and their consequences. Unpublished doctoral dissertation, Miami Institute of Psychology of the Caribbean, Center for Advanced Studies.

Greenberg, J.D. (1985). Attitudes of physicians who treat infertility toward record keeping and follow-up in the process of artificial insemination by donor. Unpublished master's thesis, University of California, Irvine.

Guinan, M.E. (1995). Artificial insemination by donor: Safety and secrecy. The Journal of the American Medical Association, 273(11), 890.

Gunning, J., & Szoke, H. (2003, June). The regulation of assisted reproductive technology. Hampshire, England and Burlington, Vermont: Ashgate Publishing.

Guttormsen, G. (1993). Familial relations in connection with donor insemination. Psychological effects of secretiveness. Tidsskr Nor Laegeforen, 113(22), 2824-2826.

Haimes, E. (1993, August). Secrecy and openness in donor insemination: A sociological comment on Daniels and Taylor. Politics and the Life Sciences, p. 178-179.

Haimes, E., & Weiner, K. (2000, July). 'Everybody's got a dad...'. Issues for lesbian families in the management of donor insemination. Sociology of Health & Illness, 22(4), 477-499.

Halliwell, R. (2003, May 16). Discovering my father was an anonymous sperm donor ruined by childhood. The Daily Mail, p. 34.

Hanson, A. (2001, September). Donor insemination: Eugenic and feminist implications. Medical Anthropology Quarterly, 15(3), 287.

Hargreaves, K. (2006, April). Constructing families and kinship through donor insemination. Sociology of Health & Illness, 28(3), 261-283.

Harrison, M. (1995). Reproductive technology and ethics in child and adolescent psychiatry. Child & Adolescent Psychiatric Clinics of North America, 4(4), 837-852.

Hassiakos, D., Zourlas, P.A., & Mantzavinos, T. (1990). Artificial insemination with fresh donor semen. International Journal of Fertility, 35(5), 292.

He donated sperm. Is he a father? (2005, November 26). The New York Times, p. A14.

Herman, R. (1992, February 11). When the 'father' is a sperm donor: A new look at secrecy. Washington Post, p. WH10.

Herz, E.K. (1989). Infertility and bioethical issues of the new reproductive technologies. Psychiatric Clinics of North America, 12(1), 117-131.

Hill, D. (1992, February). Doing business at the sperm bank—how to deposit, how to withdraw. Cosmopolitan, 212(2), 208.

Hirschman, E.C. (1991). Babies for sale: Market ethics and the new reproductive technologies. Journal of Consumer Affairs, 25(2), 358.

History of reproduction evolution and the role of man. (1998, December 20). The New Straits Times Press, p. 12, New Sunday Times, p. 2.

Hitchens, D.J. (1984). Lesbians choosing motherhood: Legal issues in donor insemination. San Francisco: Lesbian Rights Project.

Hogerzeil, H.V., Knijn, T., & Mol, B.W.J. (1996). Socio-economic characteristics of artificial insemination donor (AID) couples compared with matched population controls. European Journal of Obstetrics, Gynecology and Reproductive Biology, 64(1), 111.

Holbrook, S.M. (1996). Social workers' attitudes toward participants' rights in adoption and new reproductive technologies. Health & Social Work, 21(4), 257-266.

Holbrook, S.M. (1993/4). <u>Traditional adoptions and newer options for becoming parents: Social workers' attitudes toward the rights of various participants in adoption, donor insemination, surrogacy, and in vitro fertilization.</u> Unpublished doctoral dissertation, New York University.

Holmes, H.B. (1993). Openness, fatherhood, and responsibility: A feminist analysis. <u>Politics and the Life Sciences,</u> p. 180-182.

How it feels to be a child of donor insemination. (2002, March 30). <u>British Medical Journal, 324</u>(7340), 797.

Humphrey, M., & Humphrey, H. (1987). Marital relationships in couples seeking donor insemination. <u>Journal of Biosocial Science, 19</u>(2), 209-219.

Humphrey, M., & Humphrey, H. (1988). <u>Families with a difference: Varieties of surrogate parenthood.</u> London, England: Routledge.

Humphrey, M., Humphrey, H., & Ainsworth-Smith, I. (1991). Screening couples for parenthood by donor insemination. <u>Social Science & Medicine, 32</u>(3), 273.

Hunter, M., Salter-Ling, N., & Glover, L. (2000, November). Donor insemination: Telling children about their origins. <u>Child and Adolescent Mental Health, 5</u>(4), 157-163.

Hutton, C. (1999, November 11). Sperm donor scheme at risk. <u>The Nelson Mail; Independent Newspapers Ltd.,</u> p. 3.

ID consent donors now available; New Fairfax Cryobank program allows donor contact when offspring reach adulthood. (2006, January 24). <u>Business Wire.</u>

Ince, S., Sistare, C.T., Gibson, M., Hornstein, F., & Laqueur, T.W. (1994). <u>Living with contradictions: Controversies in feminist social ethics.</u> Boulder, CO: Westview Press. (Chapter: Contract child production, 387-429).

Ingrum, P.S. (1992). College students' attitude and schema formation for artificial/donor insemination. Unpublished master's thesis, San Diego State University.

Institute for Science Law, and Technology Working Group. (1998, July 31). ART into science: Regulation of fertility techniques. Science, 281(5377), 651-652.

Irvine, D.S., Cawood, E.H., Richardson, D.W., MacDonald, E., & Aitken, R.J. (1995). A survey of semen donation: Phase II the view of the donors. Human Reproduction, 10(10), 2752-2753.

Isaacs, Florence. (1986, February). High-tech pregnancies. Good Housekeeping, 202, 79-82.

Ison, D. (1983). Artificial insemination by donor. Bramcote: Grove.

Israeloff, R. (1994, August). Family secrets. Parents, p. 37-39.

Jackson, E. (2001, May). Regulating reproduction: Law, technology and autonomy. Oxford and Portland, Oregon: Hart Publishing.

Jansen, R., & Mortimer, D. (1999, April 15). Towards reproductive certainty: Fertility and genetics beyond 1999: The Plenary Proceedings of the 11th World Congress. New York, NY: Parthenon Publishing Group.

Janssens, P.M.W., Simons, A.H.M., van Kooij, R.J., Blokziji, E., & Dunselman, G.A.J. (2006, April 1). A new Dutch Law regulating provision of identifying information of donors to offspring: Background, content and impact. Human Reproduction, 21(4), 852-856.

Jayakrishnan, K. (1991). Experience from fresh donor insemination. Journal of Obstetrics and Gynaecology of India, 41(2), 214-218.

Jerome, L. (1987). Psychological patterns in donor insemination couples. Canadian Journal of Psychiatry, 32(4), 326.

Johnston, J. (2002, Winter). Mum's the word: Donor anonymity in assisted reproduction. <u>Health Law Review, 11</u>(1), 51.

Jones, G. (2003, January 27). Sperm donor offspring can meet father. <u>Daily Telegraph.</u>

Judgment reserved in sperm donor case. (2002, June 1). <u>British Medical Journal, 324</u>(7349), 1294.

Karow, A.M. (1993). Confidentiality and American semen donors. <u>International Journal of Fertility, 38</u>(3), 147-151.

Karow, A.M. (1992). Gamete donation and disclosure. <u>Fertility and Sterility, 57</u>(4), 943-945.

Kaufman, S.A. (1978). <u>You can have a baby: New hope for childless couples.</u> New York: Bantam Books.

Kearney, B. (1998). <u>High-tech conception: A comprehensive handbook for consumers.</u> New York: Bantam Books.

Kirkman, M. (2003, December). Parents' contributions to the narrative identity of offspring of donor-assisted conception. <u>Social Science & Medicine, 57</u>(11), 2229.

Kirkman, M. (2004, July-August). Saviours and satyrs: Ambivalence in narrative meanings of sperm provision. <u>Culture, Health & Sexuality, 6</u>(4), 319-334.

Klock, S.C. (1997). The controversy surrounding privacy or disclosure among donor gamete recipients. <u>Journal of Assisted Reproductive Genetics, 14</u>(7), 378-380.

Klock, S.C., Jacob, M.C., & Maier, D. (1996). A comparison of single and married recipients of donor insemination. <u>Human Reproduction, 11</u>(11), 2554-2557.

Klock, S.C., Jacob, M.C., & Maier, D. (1994). Donor insemination recipients: Attitudes toward disclosure and other psychological variables. Fertility and Sterility, 62 (Suppl.), 123.

Klock, S.C., Jacob, M.C., & Maier, D. (1994). A prospective study of donor insemination recipients: Secrecy, privacy, and disclosure. Fertility and Sterility, 62(3), 477.

Klock, S.C., & Maier, D. (1991). Guidelines for the provision of psychological evaluations for infertile patients at the University of Connecticut Health Center. Fertility and Sterility, 56(4), 680-685.

Klock, S.C. & Maier, D. (1991). Psychological factors related to donor insemination. Fertility and Sterility, 56, 489-495.

Knoppers, B.M. (1993). Donor insemination: Children as In Concreto or In Abstracto subjects of rights? Politics and the Life Sciences, 12(2), 182-185.

Koehler, K.E. (1996). Artificial insemination: In the child's best interest? Albany Law Journal of Science & Technology, 5(2), 321-338.

Kondro, W. (2000, January 6). On the trail of sperm-donor dads: Canada must balance competing rights to information and privacy as it joins trend toward more openness in reproductive technology. The Globe and Mail (Canada's National Newspaper). Canada.

Kovacs, D. (1997). The AID child and the alternative family: Who pays? Australian Journal of Family Law, 11(2), 141-163.

Kovacs, G.T., Morgan, G.C., Rawson, G., & Wood, C. (1986). Community attitudes to artificial insemination by donor. Australian Family Physician, 15(1), 50-51.

Kremer, J. (1996). Influence of donor insemination on sexual functions of recipients. European Journal of Obstetrics, Gynecology and Reproductive Biology, 67(2), 185.

Kremer, J., Frijling, B.W., & Nass, J.L. (1984, March 17). Psychosocial aspects of parenthood by artificial insemination donor. Lancet, 1(8377), 628.

Landau, R. (1998). Secrecy, anonymity, and deception in donor insemination: A genetic, psycho-social and ethical critique. Social Work in Health Care, 28(1), 75-89.

Lansac, J., & Royere D. (2001, February). Follow-up studies of children born after frozen sperm donation. Human Reproduction Update, 7(1), 33-37.

Lasker, J.N. (1993). Doctors and donors: A comment on secrecy and openness in donor insemination. Politics and the Life Sciences, 12(2), 186-187.

Lauritzen, P. (1993). DI's dirty little secret. Politics and the Life Sciences, 12(2), 188-189.

Ledward, R.S., Crawford, L., & Symonds, E.M. (1979). Social factors in patients for artificial insemination by donor (AID). Journal of Biosocial Science, 11(4), 473-479.

Ledward, R.S., Symonds, E.M., & Eynon, S. (1982). Social and environmental factors as criteria for success in artificial insemination by donor (AID). Journal of Biosocial Science, 14(3), 263-275.

Leeb-Lundberg, S., Kjellberg, S., & Sydsjo, G. (2006, January). Helping parents to tell their children about the use of donor insemination (DI) and determining their opinions about open-identity sperm donors. Acta Obstetricia et Gynecologica Scandinavica, 85(1), 78-81.

Leiblum, S.R. (Ed). (1997). Infertility: Psychological issues and counseling strategies. New York: John Wiley & Sons.

Leiblum, S.R., & Aviv, A.L. (1997). Disclosure issues and decisions of couples who conceived via donor insemination. Journal of Psychosomatic Obstetrics and Gynaecology, 18(4), 292-300.

Leiblum, S.R., & Barbrack, C. (1983). Artificial insemination by donor: A survey of attitudes and knowledge in medical students and infertile couples. Journal of Biosocial Science, 15(2), 165-172.

Leiblum, S.R., & Hamkins, S.E. (1992). To tell or not to tell: Attitudes of reproductive endocrinologists concerning disclosure to offspring of conception via assisted insemination by donor. Journal of Psychosomatic Obstetrics and Gynaecology, 13(4), 267-276.

Levine, J.E. (1996). Disclosure: The parental experience of couples who have had a child through donor insemination and who plan to disclose this to their child in the future. (Clinical paper, University of Wisconsin—Oshkosh).

Lifton, B.J. (1994). Journey of the adopted self: A quest for wholeness. New York: HarperCollins.

Liljestrand, P. (1990). Rhetoric and reason donor insemination politics in Sweden. Unpublished doctoral dissertation, University of California, San Francisco.

Lorbach, C. (2003, January 1). Experiences of donor conception: Parents, offspring and donors through the years. London, England and Philadelphia, PA: Jessica Kingsley Publishers.

Lui, S.C., Weaver, S.M., Robinson, J., Debono, M., Nieland, M., Killick, S.R., & Hay, D.M. (1995). A survey of semen donor attitudes. Human Reproduction, 10(1), 234-238.

Lycett, E., Daniels, K., Curson, R., & Golombok, S. (2005, March 1). School-aged children of donor insemination: A study of parents' disclosure patterns. Human Reproduction, 20(3), 810-819.

MacDonald, R. (2002, March 30). Children of donor insemination. British Medical Journal, 324(7340), 796.

MacDougall, K., Becker, G., Scheib, J.E., & Nachtigall, R.D. (2007, March). Strategies for disclosure: How parents approach telling their children that they were conceived with donor gametes. <u>Fertility and Sterility, 87</u>(3), 524.

Macintyre, S., & Sooman, A. (1991). Non-paternity and prenatal genetic screening. <u>The Lancet, 338</u>(8771), 869.

Mahlstedt, P.P. (1994). Psychological issues of infertility and assisted reproductive technology. <u>Urologic Clinics of North America, 21</u>(3), 557-566.

Mahlstedt, P.P., & Probasco, K.A. (1991). Sperm donors: Their attitudes toward providing medical and psychosocial information for recipient couples and donor offspring. <u>Fertility and Sterility, 56</u>(4), 747-753.

Maier, T. (1997, May 4). Multiple child births from same sperm donor raise ethical concerns. <u>Ann Arbor News.</u>

Makler, A., (1995). Donor insemination according to recent and strict guidelines—How safe can patients and doctors be? <u>Human Reproduction, 10</u>(8), 2050.

Marwick, C. (1988). Artificial insemination faces regulation, testing of donor semen, other measures. <u>The Journal of the American Medical Association, 260</u>(10), 1339.

Mask, M., Mask, J.L., Hensley, J., & Craig, S.L. (1995). <u>Family secrets.</u> Nashville, TN: Thomas Nelson Publishers.

Matot, J.P., & Gustin, M.L. (1990). Filiation and secrecy in artificial insemination with donor. <u>Human Reproduction, 5</u>(5), 632-633.

Mattes, J. (2000). New SMC Sibling Registry Has Been Started. <u>Single Mothers by Choice.</u> (available on http://www.parentsplace.com)

Mattes, J. (1993). Should donor insemination information be more available? <u>Single Mothers by Choice, 44</u>, 1. (available from the Infertility Network)

McCarthy, S. (1997). Ethics of fertility treatment. Nursing Times, 93(40), 48.

McWhinnie, A. (1993). Doubts and realities in DI family relationships. Politics and the Life Sciences, 12(2), 189-191.

McWhinnie, A. (1996). Families following assisted conception: What do we tell our child? Dundee: University of Dundee, School of Social Work.

McWhinnie, A. (2000, February). Families from assisted conception: Ethical and psychological issues. Human Fertility, 3(1), 13-19.

McWhinnie, A. (2001, May). Gamete donation and anonymity. Human Reproduction, 16(5), 807-817.

McWhinnie, A. (1996). Outcome for families created by assisted conception programmes. Journal of Assisted Reproduction and Genetics, 13(4), 363-365.

McWhinnie, A. (1995). A study of parenting of IVF and DI children. Medicine & Law, 14(7-8), 501-508.

Mechanick Braverman, A. (1989). Beliefs about artificial insemination by donor as a function of selected variables. Unpublished doctoral dissertation, University of Pennsylvania.

Mechanick Braverman, A., & English, M.E. (1992). Creating brave new families with advanced reproductive technologies. NAACOGS Clinical Issues in Perinatal and Womens Health Nursing, 3(2), 353-363.

Meijer, A.M., Hamerlynck, J.V., & Schagen, S. (1980). Psychosocial aspects of donor insemination. Ned Tijdschr Geneeskd, 124(16), 592-599.

Melina, L.R. (1989). Making sense of adoption: A parent's guide: Conversations and activities for families formed through adoption, donor insemination, surrogacy, and in vitro fertilization. New York: Harper & Row.

Meltz, B.F. (1998, March 19). If you had help conceiving, don't keep it a secret. Boston globe, p. F1.

Menning, B.E. (1988). Infertility: A guide for the childless couple, second edition. New York: Prenctice Hall Press.

Meyer, H.S. (1993). Family bonds: Adoption and the politics of parenting. The Journal of the American Medical Association, 270(19), 2383. (book review)

Meyer, H.S. (1993, November 17). Stories of adoption: Loss and reunion. The Journal of the American Medical Association, 270(19), 2383. (book review)

Miall, C.E. (1989). Reproductive technology vs. the stigma of involuntary childlessness. Social Casework, 70(1), 43-50.

Micioni G., Jeker, L., de Vita, S., Bianchi, G., Zeeb, M., & Campana, A. (1985). Psychological aspects of requests for artificial insemination using a donor. Data on 740 couples. Journal de Gynecologie Obstetrique et Biologie de la Reproduction, 14(6), 695-702.

Micioni, G., Jeker, L., Zeeb, M., & Campana, A. (1987). Doubtful and negative psychological indications for A.I.D.: A study of 835 couples: Treatment outcome in couples with doubtful indication. Journal of Psychosomatic Obstetrics & Gynaecology, 6(2), 89-99.

Miller, K. (2007, February 4). Catching up; Donor's offspring find one another. Star Tribune, p. 03E.

Milsom, I., & Bergman, P. (1982). A study of parental attitudes after donor insemination (AID). Acta Obstetricia et Gynecologica Scandinavica, 61(2), 125-128.

Mises, R., Semenov, G., & Huerre, P. (1978). Psychological problems associated with artificial insemination from donor. Confrontations Psychiatriques, 16, 219-236.

Mohler, M., & Frazer, L. (2002, March 15). A donor insemination guide: Written by and for lesbian women. Binghamton, NY: Harrington Park Press.

Monarch, K.L. (1995). Mother's perception of the impact on her child as a result of his/her conception by artificial insemination by an anonymous donor. Unpublished doctoral dissertation, California State University, Long Beach.

Montuschi, O. (2000). Parenting children conceived using donated eggs or sperm: Is it different? DC Network News, (15), 3-4.

Morawski, J.G. (1998). Imaginings of parenthood: Artificial insemination, experts, gender relations, and paternity. Washington, DC: American Psychological Association.

Mulcare, S.L., & Aguinis, H. (1999). Effects of adoptive status on evaluations of children. Journal of Social Psychology, 139(2), 159-172.

Murphy, G. (2002, August 3). Donor insemination: Finding your roots. The Lancet, 360(9330), 419.

Nachtigall, R.D. (1993). Secrecy: An unresolved issue in the practice of donor insemination. American Journal of Obstetrics and Gynecology, 168(6), 1846.

Nachtigall, R.D., Becker, G., Quiroga, S.S., & Tschann, J.M. (1998). The disclosure decision: Concerns and issues of parents of children conceived through donor insemination. American Journal of Obstetrics and Gynecology, 178(6), 1165.

Nachtigall, R.D., Tschann, J.M., Szkupinski, Quiroga, S., Pitcher, L., & Becker, G. (1997). Stigma, disclosure, and family functioning among parents of children conceived through donor insemination. Fertility and Sterility, 68(1), 83-89.

Nakao, A. (1993, May 23). Who's my dad? San Francisco Chronicle, p. D1.

Nelson, P., & Kornet, A. (1995). Sperm donors: The guys who give. New Woman, 25(11), 98.

Nicholas, M.K., & Tyler, J.P. (1983). Characteristics, attitudes and personalities of AI donors. Clinical Reproduction and Fertility, 2(1), 47-54.

Nielsen, A.F., Pedersen, B., Lauritsen, J.G. (1995). Psychosocial aspects of donor insemination. Attitudes and opinions of Danish and Swedish donor insemination patients to psychosocial information being supplied to offspring and relatives. Acta Obstetricia et Gynecologica Scandinavica, 74(1), 45-50.

Nijs, P., Demyttenaere, K., & Hoppenbrouwers, L. (1986). Donor insemination, adoption, in vitro fertilization: Psychosocial and psychosexual aspects. Gynakologe, 19(1), 23-27.

Offerman-Zuckerberg, J. (1989). Gender in transition: A new frontier. New York: Plenum Medical Book Co.

Origin unknown. (1999, October 14). Sperm donors want to keep it that way. The Guardian, p. 23.

Orr, D. (2002, May 15). The moral consequences of this baby hunger; Adopted children are told their history as early as possible. Why can't donor offspring have the same rights? The Independent, p. 17.

Oskarsson, T., Dimitry, E.S., Mills, M.S., Hunt, J., & Winston, R.M. (1991). Attitudes towards gamete donation among couples undergoing in vitro fertilization. British Journal of Obstetrics and Gynaecology, 98(4), 351-356.

Overall, C. (1989). The future of human reproduction. Toronto, Ontario: The Women's Press.

Owens, D.J., Edelmann, R.E., & Humphrey, M.E. (1993). Male infertility and donor insemination: Couples' decisions, reactions and counselling needs. Human Reproduction, 8(6), 880-885.

Patrizio, P., & Mastroianni, A. (2001, October). Gamete donation and anonymity. Human Reproduction, 16(10), 2036-2038.

Paul, J., & Spencer, M. (New South Wales Infertility Social Workers Group). (1988). How I began: The story of donor insemination. Carlton, Victoria: Fertility Society of Australia.

Pederson, B., Nielsen, A.F., & Lauritsen, J.G. (1994). Psychosocial aspects of donor insemination. Sperm donors—Their motivations and attitudes to artificial insemination. Acta Obstetricia et Gynecologica Scandinavica, 73(9), 701-705.

Penick, B.R. (1998). Note—Give the child a legal father: A plea for Iowa to adopt a statute regulating artificial insemination by anonymous donor. Iowa Law Review, 83(3), 633.

Pennings, G. (1997). The internal coherence of donor insemination practice: Attracting the right type of donor without paying. Human Reproduction, 12(9), 1842.

Penochet, J.C., Moron, P., & Jarrige, A. (1979). Psychiatric complications linked to donor artificial insemination. Annales Medico-Psychologiques, 137,6-7, 635-641.

Phillips, J. (2003, March 3). Teen deserves to learn truth about his birth. The Seattle Times, p. E8.

Physician explores right to know vs. right to privacy. (1996, March 29). Knight-Ridder/Tribune News Service, p. 329K1815.

Pitrolo, E.A. (1996). The birds, the bees, and the deep freeze: Is there international consensus in the debate over assisted reproductive technologies? Houston Journal of International Law, 19(1), 147-206.

Pittaway, K. (2000, May). Secrets and lies: When it comes to donor insemination, anonymity is bad medicine. Chatelaine, p. 36.

Poteet, G.W., & Lamar, E.K. (1986). Artificial insemination by donor: Problems and issues. Health Care Women International, 7(5), 391-399.

Prattke, T.W., & Gass-Sternas, K.A. (1993). Appraisal, coping and emotional health of infertile couples undergoing donor artificial insemination. Journal of Obstetric, Gynecologic, and Neonatal Nursing: JOGNN, 22(6), 516-527.

Purdie, A., Peek, J.C., Adair, V., Graham, F., & Fisher, R. (1994). Attitudes of parents of young children to sperm donation-implications for donor recruitment. Human Reproduction, 9(7), 1355-1358.

Purdie, A., Peek, J.C., Irwin, R., Ellis, J., Graham, F.M., & Fisher, P.R. (1992). Identifiable semen donors-attitudes of donors and recipient couples. New Zealand Medical Journal, 105(927), 27-28.

Raboy, B. (1993). Secrecy and openness in donor insemination: A new paradigm. Politics and the Life Sciences, 12(2), 191-192.

Rawson, G. (1984). Human artificial insemination by donor: Some Australian perspectives. New South Wales: Advisory Committee on Human Artificial Insemination.

Reading, A.E., Sledmere, C.M., & Cox, D.N. (1982). A survey of patient attitudes towards artificial insemination by donor. Journal of Psychosomatic Research, 26(4), 429-433.

Reeves, R. (1999, July 25). Sperm donors to be traced. The Observer. (in DI Network News, Winter 1999/2000)

Reid, J. (1996). Mummy, what's a sperm donor? The Independent, (2938), p. S4(2).

Repromed. A Canadian study of disclosure. (available from the Infertility Network)

Resemblance talk difficult for parents of children conceived with donor gametes, United States. (2006, May). Reproductive Health Matters, 14(27), 211.

Richardson, C.A., Dickinson, A.S., Barratt, C.L.R., & Cooke, I.D. (1990). Using a donor insemination management system. British Medical Bulletin, 46(3), 813.

Richardson, J.W. (1987). The role of a psychiatric consultant to an artificial insemination by donor program. Psychiatric Annals, 17(2), 101-105.

Riordan, T. (1994). The threat of donor insemination. New York: Focal Point & Resolve. (available from the Infertility Network)

Robertson, J.A. (1994). Children of choice: Freedom and the new reproductive technologies. Princeton, NJ: Princeton University Press.

Robertson, J.A. (1995). Ethical and legal issues in human embryo donation. Fertility and Sterility, 64(5), 885-894.

Robinson, J.N., Forman, R.G., Clark, A.M., Egan, D.M., Chapman, M.G., & Barlow, D.H. (1991). Attitudes of donors and recipients to gamete donation. Human Reproduction, 6, 307-309.

Rodocker, M.M. (1989). A follow-up study of couples who have successfully completed donor insemination. Unpublished doctoral dissertation, Professional School of Psychology. (Available from University Microfilms, Ann Arbor, MI).

Rojo-Moreno, J., Valdemoro, C., Garcia-Merita, M.L., & Tortajada, M. (1996). Analysis of the attitudes and emotional processes in couples undergoing artificial insemination by donor. Human Reproduction, 11(2), 294.

Roman, M.B. (1993, January). Breaking the genetic silence. Lear's, 5, 37-38.

Rose. Australian Psychologist, 14(5), 1392.

Rose, J. (1999). The response of an adult donor insemination offspring to the article "The psychology of assisted reproduction—or psychology assisting its reproduction?" Australian Psychologist, 34(3), 220.

Rosenberg, G., & Weissman, A. (2006, December 13). International social health care policy, program, and studies (Social work in health care). Binghamton, NY: Haworth Press.

Rosenkvist, H. (1981). Donor insemination: A prospective socio-psychiatric investigation of 48 couples. Danish Medical Bulletin, 28(4), 133-148.

Rosenthal, M.S. (1995). The fertility sourcebook. Los Angeles: Lowell House.

Rowland, R. (1983). Attitudes and opinions of donors on an artificial insemination by donor (AID) programme. Clinical Reproductive Fertility, 2(4), 249-259.

Rowland, R. (1993). Donor insemination to in vitro fertilization: The confusion grows. Politics and the Life Sciences, p. 192.

Rowland, R. (1985). The social and psychological consequences of secrecy in artificial insemination by donor (AID) programmes. Social Science & Medicine, 21(4), 391-396.

Rubin, B. (1965). Psychological aspects of human artificial insemination. Archives of General Psychiatry, 13(2), 121-132.

Rumball, A., & Adair, V. (1999). Telling the story: Parents' scripts for donor offspring. Human Reproduction, 14(5), 1392-1399.

Salter-Ling N., Hunter, M., & Glover, L. (2001, August 17). Donor insemination: Exploring the experience of treatment and intention to tell. Journal of Reproductive and Infant Psychology, 19(3), 175-186.

Sanchagrin, M.L., Humber, E.B., Speirs, C.C., & Duder, S. (1993). A survey of Quebec pediatrician's attitudes toward donor insemination. Clinical Pediatrics, 32(4), 226.

Sauer, M.V., Gorrill, M.F., Zeffer, K.B., & Bustillo, M. (1989). Attitudinal survey of sperm donors to an artificial insemination clinic. Journal of Reproductive Medicine, 34(5), 362-364.

Sauer, M.V., Rodi, I.A., Scrooc, M., Bustillo, M., & Buster, J.E. (1988). Survey of attitudes regarding the use of siblings for gamete donation. Fertility and Sterility, 49(4), 721-722.

Savage, O.M. Njikam. (1992). Artificial donor insemination in Yaounde: Some socio-cultural considerations. Social Science and Medicine, 35(7), 907.

Savage, O.M. Njikam. (1995). Secrecy still the best policy: Donor insemination in Cameroon. Politics and the Life Sciences: The Journal of the Association for Politics and the Life Sciences, 14(1), 87.

Scheib, J.E. (1996/7). The psychology of female choice in the context of donor insemination. Unpublished doctoral dissertation, McMaster University, Canada.

Scheib, J.E., Riordan, M., & Rubin, S. (2005, January 1). Adolescents with open-identity sperm donors: Reports from 12-17 year olds. Human Reproduction, 20(1), 239-252.

Scheib, J.E., Riordan, M., & Rubin, S. (2003, May). Choosing identity-release sperm donors: The parents' perspective 13-18 years later. Human Reproduction, 18(5), 1115-1127.

Schilling, G. (1995). Family secrets exemplified by heterologous insemination. Psychotherapie, Psychosomatik, Medizinische Psychologie, 45(1), 16-23.

Schilling, G. (2001, October). Reproductive epidemiology. Secrecy and openness in donor offspring. Human Reproduction, 16(10), 2244-2245.

Schilling, G., & Conrad, R. (2003, August). Parental assessment of children conceived by artificial donor insemination-possible ways to reduce cognitive dissonance. Journal of Psychosomatic Research, 55(2), 144.

Schnitter, J.T. (1995). Let me explain: A story about donor insemination. Indianapolis, IN: Perspectives Press.

Schooler, J. (1995). Searching for a past: The adopted adult's unique process of finding identity. Colorado Springs, CO: Pinon Press.

Schover, L.R. Collins, R.L., & Richards, S. (1992). Psychological aspects of donor insemination: Evaluation and follow-up of recipient couples. Fertility and Sterility, 57(3), 583-590.

Schover, L.R., Greenhalgh, L.F., Richards, S.I., & Collins, R.L. (1994). Psychological screening and the success of donor insemination. Human Reproduction, 9(1), 176-178.

Schover, L.R., Rothmann, S.A., & Collins, R.L. (1992). The personality and motivation of semen donors: A comparison with oocyte donors. Human Reproduction, 7(4), 575-579.

Schutte, M. (1987). Reform of the legal position of illegitimate children with particular reference to the status of children conceived by artificial fertilisation. Unpublished doctoral dissertation, University of South Africa, South Africa.

The secret life of families: Truth-telling, privacy, and reconciliation in a tell-all society. (1998, February 16). Publishers Weekly, 245(7), 197. (book review)

Seligson, S.V. (1995). Seeds of doubt: A successful donor insemination service catering to heterosexual single women and lesbians raises some difficult questions. The Atlantic Monthly, 275(3), 28.

Shenfield, F. (1994). Particular requests in donor insemination: Comments on the medical duty of care and the welfare of the child. Human Reproduction, 9(11), 1976.

Singer, D., & Hunter, M. (2003, March 1). Assisted human reproduction: Psychological and ethical dilemmas. London, England and Philadelphia, PA: Whurr Publisher Ltd.

Singer, E. Talking with children conceived through DI, egg donor or surrogacy. Resolve. (available from the Infertility Network)

Skjaeraasen, J. (1993). Donor insemination-openness or secretiveness? Tidsskr Nor Laegeforen, 113(22), 2791.

Slover, S.L. (1989). Third party conception: The ambivalent solution. Infertility Awareness, 5(6), 1,3.

Smith, H.J. (1996). My parent(s) made me in a special way: With love and the help of donor insemination. Ladysmith, BC: H.J. Smith.

Smith, J. (1999, July 30). Comment and analysis: Daddies and donors. The Guardian, p. 18.

Snowden, R. (1997). Implications counselling for couples considering donor insemination. Sheffield, UK: BICA Publications.

Snowden, R. (1993). Sharing information about DI in the UK. Politics and the Life Sciences, p. 194.

Snowden, R., & Mitchell, G.D. (1983). The artificial family: A consideration of artificial insemination by donor. London: Unwin Paperacks.

Snowden, R., & Snowden, E.M. (1993). The gift of a child: A guide to donor insemination. Exeter, UK: University of Exeter Press.

Society of Obstetricians & Gynaecologists. Ethical considerations of NRTs: Gamete/pre-embryo donor's consents, banking & handling of gametes & embryos. (available from the Infertility Network)

Solberg, C. (1997). Stork market: Fertility clinics enjoy a baby boom. Corporate Report-Minnesota, 28(10), 70.

Son must know his real parents: Dear Deidre. (2005, May 14). The Sun, p. 41.

Sorosky, A. Lessons from the adoption experience: Anticipating times of developmental conflict for the ART child. (available from the Infertility Network)

South Australia. Parliament. Legislative Council. Select Committee on Artificial Insemination by Donor, In-Vitro Fertilization and Embryo Transfer Procedures and Related Matters in South Australia. (1987). Report of the Select Committee of the Legislative Council on artificial insemination by donor, in-vitro fertilization and embryo transfer procedures and related matters in South Australia. Adelaide, Australia: Government Printer.

South Australia. Working Party on In Vitro Fertilization and Artificial Insemination by Donor. (1984). Report of the Working Party on in vitro fertilization and artificial insemination by donor. Adelaide, Australia: South Australian Health Commission.

Spallone, P., & Steinberg, D.L. (1987). Made to order: The myth of reproductive and genetic progress. Oxford: Pergamon Press.

Sperm banks and clinics: Where to go and what to know. (1994, March). Washingtonian, 29, 114.

Sperm donor father calls offspring. (2007, February 14). The Evening Standard, p. 4.

Stein, M. (1994, September 20). Making babies or playing god? Startling new developments in reproductive technology are raising serious ethical, legal and religious questions. Family Circle, 107(13), 67.

Stewart, C.R., Daniels, K.R., & Boulnois, J.D.H. (1982). The development of a psychosocial approach to artificial insemination of donor sperm. New Zealand Medical Journal, 95(721), 853-856.

Stiffler, L.H. (1992). Synchronicity & reunion: The genetic connection of adoptees & birthparents. Hobe Sound, FL: FEA Publishing.

Tadir, M. (1994). The "silent third party": An exploratory research in gamete donation. Unpublished doctoral dissertation, United States International University.

Templeton, A. (1991). Gamete donation and anonymity. British Journal of Obstetrics and Gynaecology, 98(4), 343-345.

Teper, S., & Symonds, E.M. (1983). Artificial insemination by donor: Problems and perspectives. Proceedings of the Annual Symposium of the Eugenics Society, 19, 19-52.

Thepot, F., Mayaux, M.J., Czyglick, F., & Wack, T. (1996). Incidence of birth defects after artificial insemination with frozen donor spermatozoa: A collaborative study of the French CECOS Federation on 11,535 pregnancies. Human Reproduction, 11(10), 2319.

Thorn, P., & Daniels, K. (2003, February). A group-work approach in family building by donor insemination: Empowering the marginalized. Human Fertility, 6(1), 46-50.

Triseliotis, J. Donor insemination and the child. (available from the Infertility Network)

Turner, A.J. (2000, September). Psychology. What does it mean to be a donor offspring? The identity experiences of adults conceived by donor insemination and the implications for counselling and therapy. Human Reproduction, 15(9), 2041-2051.

Turner, C. A call for openness in donor insemination.

Tyler, J.P., Nicholas, M.K., Crockett, N.G., & Driscoll, G.L. (1983). Some attitudes to artificial insemination by donor. Clinical Reproduction and Fertility, 2(2), 151-160.

Ubelacker, S. (1993, August). Brave new womb. Chatelaine, 66(8), 30.

van Berkel, D., van der Veen, L., Kimmel, I., & te Velde, E. (1999). Male factor—Differences in the attitudes of couples whose children were conceived through artificial insemination by donor in 1980 and in 1996. Fertility and Sterility, 71(2), 226-231.

van den Akker, O. (2006, March 15). A review of family donor constructs: Current research and future directions. Human Reproduction Update, 12(2), 91-101.

Vanfraussen, K., & Ponjaert-Kristoffersen, I. (2001, September). Psychology and counselling. An attempt to reconstruct children's donor concept: A comparison between children's and lesbian parents' attitudes towards donor anonymity. Human Reproduction, 16(9), 2019-2025.

Van Hall, E.V. (1985). The gynaecologist and artificial reproduction. Journal of Psychosomatic Obstetrics & Gynaecology, 4(4), 317-320.

van Zyl, L. (2002). Intentional parenthood and the nuclear family. Journal of Medical Humanities, 23(2), 107-118.

Varley, N. (1999, August 12). The sperm donor. The Times, p. 37.

Vega Gutierrez, M. (1992). Valoracion bioetica y medico-legal de la reproduccion asistida en la comunidad europea y su repercusion en los derechol del nino; A bioethical and medicolegal evaluation of assisted human reproduction in the EC and its implications for the rights of the child. Unpublished doctoral dissertation, Universidad de Valladolid, Spain.

Vercollone, C.F., Moss, H., & Moss, R. (1997). Helping the stork: The choices and challenges of donor insemination. New York: Macmillan.

Vergin, L.A. (1981). Infertility: A guide for pastoral care and counseling. Unpublished doctoral dissertation, School of Theology at Claremont.

Vernaeve, V., Festre, V., Baetens, P., Devroey, P., Van Steirteghem, A., & Tournaye, H. (2005, February). Reproductive decisions by couples undergoing artificial insemination with donor sperm for severe male infertility: Implications for medical counselling. International Journal of Andrology, 28(1), 22-26.

Verrier, N.N. (1993). The primal wound: Understanding the adopted child. Baltimore: Gateway Press.

Victoria. Committee to Consider the Social, Ethical, and Legal Issues Arising from In Vitro Fertilization. (1986). The Committee to Consider the Social, Ethical, and Legal Issues Arising from In Vitro Fertilization. Melbourne: The Committee to Consider the Social, Ethical, and Legal Issues Arising from In Vitro Fertilization.

Victoria. Committee to Consider the Social, Ethical, and Legal Issues Arising from In Vitro Fertilization. (1983). Issue paper on donor gametes in IVF. Melbourne: The Committee to Consider the Social, Ethical, and Legal Issues Arising from In Vitro Fertilization.

Victoria. Committee to Consider the Social, Ethical, and Legal Issues Arising from In Vitro Fertilization. (1984). Issue paper on donor gametes in IVF. Melbourne: The Committee to Consider the Social, Ethical, and Legal Issues Arising from In Vitro Fertilization.

Victoria. Committee to Consider the Social, Ethical, and Legal Issues Arising from In Vitro Fertilization. (1983). Report on donor gametes in IVF. Melbourne: The Committee to Consider the Social, Ethical, and Legal Issues Arising from In Vitro Fertilization.

Victoria. Committee to Consider the Social, Ethical, and Legal Issues Arising from In Vitro Fertilization. (1984). Report on donor gametes in IVF: The status of the children born as a result of donor gametes in IVF. Melbourne: The Committee to Consider the Social, Ethical, and Legal Issues Arising from In Vitro Fertilization.

Victory in hunt for dads. (2002, July 27). The Sun, p. 27.

Walker, A., Gregson, S., & McLaughlin, E. (1987). Attitudes towards donor insemination-A post-Warnock survey. Human Reproduction, 2(8), 745-750.

Waltzer, H. (1981). Anonymity and donor insemination. <u>American Journal of Psychiatry, 138</u>(2), 262.

Waltzer, H. (1982). Psychological and legal aspects of artificial insemination (A.I.D.): An overview. <u>American Journal of Psychotherapy, 36</u>(1), 91-102.

Warnock U-turn on naming sperm donors. (2002, May 13). <u>The Guardian,</u> p. 6.

Wavell, S. (1997, July 6). A donor father's sins of omission. <u>The Sunday Times,</u> p. N6.

Weaver, E. (1998). Private choices, public consequences: A personal look at how reproductive technology has affected the legal, moral, and ethical decisions we make about life. <u>Library Journal, 123</u>(3), 166. (book review)

Wedeward, T.J. (1987). <u>Stressors, appraisal, coping, and emotional health status of couples undergoing artificial insemination with donor semen.</u> Unpublished master's thesis, University of Wisconsin, Madison.

Weil, E. (1997). Privacy and disclosure: The psychological impact on gamete donors and recipients in assisted reproduction. <u>Journal of Assisted Reproductive Genetics, 14</u>(7), 369-371.

Wells, S.A. (1996). <u>Michigan law for everyone.</u> Royal Oak, MI: LAWells Publishing.

Wendland, C.L., Byrn, F., & Hill, C. (1996). Donor insemination: A comparison of lesbian couples, heterosexual couples and single women. <u>Fertility and Sterility, 65</u>(4), 764.

Western Australia. Committee to Enquire into the Social, Legal and Ethical Issues Relating to In Vitro Fertilization and Its Supervision. (1986). <u>Report of the committee appointed by the Western Australian government to enquire into the social, legal and ethical issues relating to</u>

in vitro fertilization and its supervision. Perth, Western Australia: Health Department of Western Australia.

Western Australian Reproductive Technology Council. (1994). Questions and answers about the donation of human reproductive material: Donor insemination and sperm donation, donated eggs, and donated embryos. East Perth, Western Australia: Western Australian Reproductive Technology Council.

Western Australian Reproductive Technology Council. (1995). Questions and answers about the donation of human reproductive material: Donor insemination and sperm donation, donated eggs, and donated embryos. East Perth, Western Australia: Western Australian Reproductive Technology Council.

Western Australian Reproductive Technology Council. (1994). Questions and answers about donor insemination. East Perth, Western Australia: Western Australian Reproductive Technology Council.

Whither human donor insemination in Britain? (1982, March 6). Lancet, 1(8271), 545-546.

Who's my biological daddy? Children of anonymous sperm donors. (2005, June 7). Asia Africa Intelligence Wire.

Wikler, D. (1995). Policy issues in donor insemination. Stanford Law & Policy Review, 6(2), 47.

Wilcox, W.B. (2005, December 12). Who's your daddy? There's more to fatherhood than donating DNA. The Weekly Standard, 11(13).

Wilkinson, H.S. Birth is more than once: The inner world of adopted Korean children. Unpublished doctoral dissertation, Saybrook Institute, San Francisco.

Wilson, S.M. (1995). Should children conceived through the use of donor insemination have access to biographical information concerning the donor? Unpublished doctoral dissertation, McGill University, Canada.

Winkler, R.C.., Brown, D.W., Van Keppel, M., & Blanchard, A. (1988). Clinical practice in adoption. Oxford, England: Pergamon Press.

Winston, R. (1999, July 26). This foolish threat to the gift of life. Daily Mail. (available in DI Network News, Winter 1999/2000)

Wood, C. (1980). Artificial insemination by donor. Melbourne: Monash University.

Worthington, C. (1997, August). Am I selfish? Am I entitled? Am I crazy? Harper's Bazaar, (3429), 50.

Wright, K., & Richardson, S. (1998). Human in the age of mechanical reproduction. Discover, 19(5), 74.

Zolbrod, A. (1987, November). Decision making in male infertility. (available from the Infertility Network)

Zolbrod, A. (1988). The emotional distress of the artificial insemination patient. Medical Psychotherapy, 1, 161-172.

Zolbrod, A. Opinion of DI: Don't confuse secrecy with privacy. (available from the Infertility Network)

Zoldbrod, A.P. (1999). Recipient counseling for donor insemination. New York: Parthenon.

Zorn, J.R. (1996). About the HFEA patients' guide to donor insemination and in-vitro fertilization (IVF) clinics—are we crossing the rubicon? Human Reproduction, 11(7), 1367.

APPENDIX B
SUPPORT ORGANIZATIONS

Alliance for Donor Insemination Families, Inc., 9678 East Arapahoe Road, No. 143, Englewood, Colorado 80112-3703. Phone: 303-220-8400. E-mail: AllianceDI@aol.com. Leader: Susan Hollander. A nonprofit organization, the only one of its kind in the USA offering counseling, support, and information to people who are thinking of building their families using donor egg or sperm, or people who already have their donor children. Support includes assistance with how to tell children about their conception.

The Donor Conception Network, PO Box 265, Sheffield, England, S3 7YX. Phone: 44-20-8245-4369. E-mail: w.merricks@appleonline. net or olivia.m@appleonline.net. Website: www.dcnetwork.org. Leaders: Walter Merricks & Olivia Montuschi.

Originated in 1983 in the UK as DI Network, with members from UK, North America, Europe, and elsewhere. It includes those who are still coming to a decision about donated gamete treatment, those undergoing treatment, and those who already have children. Members include married and unmarried couples, single women, lesbian couples, parents who have separated, divorced, or widowed, and adults who are donor offspring.

The Donor Conception Support Group of Australia, PO Box 53, George's Hall, NSW 2198, Australia. E-mail: warrenh@ozemail.com. au. Website: www.ozemail.com.au/~warrenh. Leaders: Warren & Leonie Hewitt.

Membership consists of people considering or using donor sperm, eggs, or embryo, those who already have children conceived on donor programs, adult donor offspring, and donors, social workers, doctors, and clinic staff. DCSG believes that donor gamete families need an ongoing support system beyond the initial decision making and treatment.

Services include information, contacts, consumer advocacy, meetings and social events.

Donor Sibling Registry, PO Box 1571, Nederland CO 80466. Website: www.donorsiblingregistry.com. Email: burlwindow741@yahoo. com. Leaders: Wendy and Ryan Kramer.

The focus of the Donor Sibling Registry (DSR) is to assist individuals conceived as a result of sperm, egg or embryo donation who are seeking to make mutually desired contact with others with whom they share genetic ties.

Infertility Network, 160 Pickering Street, Toronto, Ontario, Canada, M4E 3J7. Phone: 416-691-3611. Fax: 416-690-8015. Email: DianeAllen@ InfertilityNetwork.org. Website: www.infertilitynetwork.org. Executive Director: Diane Allen.

Started in 1990 and now registered as a Canadian health charity. The goal is to provide information and support so that people can make informed choices about their family-building options. Services include referral, information, seminars, support groups.

The New Reproductive Alternatives Society, 641 Cadogan Street, Nenaimo, British Columbia, Canada V9S 1T6. Phone: 250-754-3900. E-mail: spratten@nisa.net. Leader: Shirley Pratten.

Canada's first support group for donor conceived families. Provides support, and liaison with the provincial and federal governments to work on bringing legislation that will primarily protect the needs and rights of the resulting offspring.

PCVAI internet support group. PCVAI@yahoogroups.com.

This is an internet support group for "persons conceived via artificial insemination". Leader: Bill Cordray.

Southwestern Ontario Donor Family Support Group, Reproductive Endocrinology and Infertility Program, London Health Sciences Centre, 339 Windermere Road, Ontario, Canada. N6A 5A5. Phone: 519-685-8300, ext. 32405. E-mail: jean.haase@lhsc.on.ca. Leader: Jean Haase, MSW.

Support group for those who have built their families through donated sperm or eggs, for donor conceived offspring, gamete donors, or professionals directly involved in gamete donations. Services include meetings, picnics, information.

Southwestern Ontario Network of Infertility Counsellors (SONIC).
E-mail: sfranz@pathcom.com. Facilitator: Sherry Franz.
For mental health professionals whose primary focus is infertility and reproductive health counseling.

APPENDIX C
INSTRUCTIONS TO RESEARCH PARTICIPANTS

Date _____

Dear _____,

Thank you for your interest in and agreeing to participate in this research for my Masters in Humanistic and Clinical Psychology thesis on the experience of confronting the reality of being a donor offspring. I value the unique contribution that you can make to my study and I look forward to working with you.

The purpose of this letter is to explain, in a formal way, the nature of the research design I am using, its purpose, and process, and what I am hoping you will be able to share with me. I have enclosed the Participation Release Agreement form. Please sign this and return to me in the enclosed SASE. After I receive the signed Participation Release Agreement form, we can begin the interviewing process.

Your confidentiality is important in this project. On the Participation Release Agreement form, you may select your preference for use of your real name or a fictitious name for this research report and any publications derived from it.

The research model I am using is a qualitative one, which seeks comprehensive descriptions of your experience of confronting the reality of being a donor offspring. In order for you to understand the part that I am asking you to play as a co-researcher, please consider the following commitments to the study:

1)   Before the interview, reflect upon experiences when you have confronted the reality of being a donor offspring. This includes times when you have explored internally the meaning of being a donor offspring, reached out and contacted others about your experience as a donor offspring, shared your story and concerns

with others, sought support, or other significant activities you have been involved in related to being a donor offspring.

2) An interview of approximately one to two hours in length at a mutually agreed upon time, when uninterrupted, private time is available. In person interviews are preferable, but if not possible, telephone interviews will be conducted.

3) A possible shorter follow-up interview to clarify information from the first interview.

4) These interviews will be audio-recorded in order that I may transcribe them for the purposes of delineating data for the research study.

Before our interview, please think about and recall specific episodes, situations, or events when you faced the reality of being a donor offspring, e.g. when you were told about it, when you spoke with others about it, when you were processing the experience yourself, when you acted out in more public ways related to being a donor offspring. I am seeking vivid, accurate, and comprehensive portrayals of what these experiences were like for you: your thoughts, feelings, body sensations, and behaviors, as well as situations, events, places, and people connected with your experience. This will be the basis for our interview.

Thank you for your commitment of time and energy in the participation of this research project. If you have any questions about the nature of my research before signing the release form, or if you have any concerns or would like to talk further about your experiences, please call me. I look forward to our discussions.

With warm regards,

Lynne W. Spencer

APPENDIX D
PARTICIPATION RELEASE AGREEMENT

I agree to participate in the research study "What is the experience of confronting the reality of being a donor offspring?" I understand the purpose and nature of this study and I am participating voluntarily. I grant permission for the data to be used in the process of completing a Masters in Humanistic and Clinical Psychology degree, including a thesis report, and any other future publication of the research results. I understand that a brief synopsis of each participant, including myself, will be used and will include the following information: fictitious name, age, age of being informed of being a donor offspring, circumstances of finding out about being a donor offspring, number of siblings and relationship, and other pertinent information that will help the reader come to know and recall each participant. I grant permission for the above personal information to be used. I agree to meet in person or speak on the phone for approximately one to two hours at a mutually agreed upon time and place. I grant permission for audio-tape-recording of the interview. I also agree to a shorter follow-up interview for clarification of information if necessary.

_____   _____

Research Participant   Date

_____   _____

Researcher   Date

APPENDIX E
THANK YOU LETTER AND SECOND RELEASE
AGREEMENT

May 7, 2000

Dear Research Participant,

Thank you for participating in an interview for my qualitative research on "What is the experience of confronting the reality of being a donor offspring?" Some of the participants have requested that their real names be used in the publication of this research. With donor insemination, issues of secrecy and disclosure are central and some of the participants expressed their preference for disclosure in their discussions of being a donor offspring.

As a result, I have spoken further with my thesis adviser about this issue of using real versus fictitious names in a research project. We sought standards of ethical practice in the "Ethical Principles of Psychologists and Code of Conduct" and my advisor spoke with another thesis advisor at The Center for Humanistic Studies. The result of this is that it is ethical to use real names in research if any limitation to confidentiality is done with written, informed consent from the participant.

I will describe the structure of my thesis presentation in regard to information from research participants. At the end of the research will be a list of participants, with a short description of each participant. This will include current age, age and general circumstances of finding out about being a donor offspring, and country of conception. If you choose to keep your information confidential, then this information will be adjusted to attempt to keep your identity confidential. There are a limited number of donor offspring aware of their identities and outspoken about it, so our identities are sometimes easily discovered even from limited information. I will make every effort to keep your information confidential if you desire anonymity.

Within the body of the research presentation, I will discuss themes which were derived from the interviews of donor offspring. For each theme, I will present quotes from research participants. The quotes will be presented as a group and not associated with a particular individual.

My master's thesis will be kept in the library at The Center for Humanistic Studies and may occasionally be checked out through interlibrary loan. I also hope to get parts of this information published in journal and/or book form.

Please indicate below if you would like your information kept confidential or if you prefer to use your real name in the publications of this research on "What is the experience of confronting the reality of being a donor offspring?" If you prefer to use your real name, please print it as you would like it to appear in publication. If I don't hear back from you by May 31, 2000, then I will keep your information confidential and assign a fictitious name for you.

If you have any questions about the nature of the publication of your interview information, please contact me. My goal is to present this information with the fullest respect of your wishes regarding confidentiality as a donor offspring.

Thank you for your participation! When I have completed my thesis (June/July), I will send you a summary of the findings. I hope this information helps to broaden available information regarding the lives of donor offspring.

With warm regards,

Lynne W. Spencer

In publications from the master's thesis research on "What is the experience of confronting the reality of being a donor offspring?", I request:

SPERM DONOR OFFSPRING:

A fictitious name and nonidentifying information _____

To use my real name as follows:_____
                  (write name as you would like it to appear in publication)

_____   _____

Participant signature   Date

_____   _____

Researcher signature   Date

APPENDIX F
GUIDING RESEARCH QUESTIONS

Biographical data:

1) Name
2) Age
3) Age at which informed of being a donor offspring
4) Circumstances of being informed of being a donor offspring
5) Number of siblings and relationship (i.e. donor offspring, adopted, biological, etc.)
6) Other pertinent biographical information

Guiding questions for research:

Take a moment to take a deep breath and relax. Visualize a significant time when you were actively confronting the reality of being a donor offspring (for example, processing this information yourself, sharing with others about it, seeking support, speaking out publicly, etc.)

1) Describe your experience in detail.
2) Describe the emotions you were feeling at that time.
3) What thoughts did you have during or related to this time?
4) What bodily sensations did you experience during or related to this?
5) What were your actions?
6) How did this experience involve you with other people?

Are there other times when confronting the reality of being a donor offspring were significant for you? If yes, describe this time (look at 1-6 again).

APPENDIX G
DESCRIPTION OF RESEARCH PARTICIPANTS

(1)   Bill Cordray

Age: 54
Age informed: 37

Circumstances of being informed:
    After death of younger brother, one year after death of father.
    Mother told him after he said he had thought that his dad wasn't
    really his father.

Sibling relationships:
    Brother, adopted, 4 years older.
    Brother, donor offspring, different donor, 2 years younger.
    Brother, donor offspring, different donor, 8 years younger.

(2)   Greg Wiatt

Age: 44
Age informed: 28

Circumstances of being informed:
    On his 28th birthday. Counselors told his mom the whole picture
    of Greg was wrong. He was intelligent, gifted, but he wasn't able
    to put his life together. Mom told the counselors, who advised
    her to tell Greg.

Sibling relationships:
    Two sisters, adopted.

(3)   Remington O. Schmidt ("Ted")

Age: 57
Age informed: 35

Circumstances of being informed:

On his 35th birthday. He was visiting his mother. She said she didn't want to go to her grave with this secret, and she was reacting to her husband divorcing her.

Sibling relationships:

Brother, donor offspring, 13 months younger.
Brother, donor offspring, 4 or 5 years younger.
Brother, donor offspring, 7 years younger.
Sister, adopted, 14 years younger.
(Ted believes the brothers probably all had different donors).

(4)   Rhonda (not her real name)

Age: 50's
Age informed: 40's

Circumstances of being informed:

Her mother was visiting her. Mother asked for her husband to be there, and handed her a note with all of the details. Her dad had died four years earlier and her mother had been trying to tell her since then.

Sibling relationships:

Sister, donor offspring, different donor.

(5)   Tammy (not her real name)

Age: 39
Age informed: 32

Circumstances of being informed:
   After father's death. He had wanted it kept secret.
   After he died, mom decided it was the right time to
   tell her.

Sibling relationships:
   Sister, donor offspring, same donor, 3 years older.

(6)   Sondra (not her real name)

Age informed: teens

Circumstances of being informed:
   She sensed something was not right between her and her father.
   She asked her mother if her father was actually her father. She
   told her mother that it was her right to know. Her mother told
   her.

Sibling relationships:
   Sister, donor offspring.
   Sister, biological offspring of her parents.

(7)   Janice Stevens Botsford

Age: 52
Age informed: 22

Circumstances of being informed:
> Father had died earlier that year. Mother was an honest person and was uncomfortable with keeping the secret. Mother wrestled with feeling loyal to father's wishes and having her own relationship with children, and she decided to tell them.

Sibling relationships:
> Brother, donor offspring, same donor, 4-1/2 years younger.

(8)   Barry Stevens

Age: 48
Age informed: 18

Circumstances of being informed:
> Father died earlier that year. Mother always wanted to tell them and she did. The main motivation was that she just felt she should tell them. She's a good hearted, honest person.

Sibling relationships:
> Sister, donor offspring, same donor, 4 years older.